Mother, Nurse and Infant

A Manual Especially Adapted for the Guidance of Mothers and Monthly Nurses

Vol. I

S. P. Sackett

CHAPTER I.
CONDUCT OF THE MOTHER BEFORE AND AFTER MARRIAGE.

The physical treatment of children should begin, as far as may be practicable, with the earliest formation of the embryo. It will involve the conduct of the female even before her marriage, as well as during her pregnancy—the various contingencies which effect her in health as well as in disease. Very much depends on her to insure for her child a vigorous constitution, or to prevent a feeble frame in the child. She should not *enter* into the holy state of marriage with heedless haste; if she does, she will discharge its duties with inexcusable neglect. To constitute a mother, in the best sense of the term, requires a patient endurance of fatigue, and anxious solicitude, which will sorely tax the mother's strength. I would, if possible, diminish the toil and danger of childbirth, and relieve the fatigue and anxiety of nursing.

And let me, in one paragraph, give a hint to the husband: that the responsibility and care of the children is too much laid on the mother; she is overburdened. Let the father partake in the arduous and responsible duty of their education. And let me hint, also, that the health and strength of the child depends upon the father as well as the mother.

MARRIAGE SHOULD NOT BE AT TOO EARLY A PERIOD OF LIFE.—I am not disposed to discourage early marriage, but I am decidedly opposed to a premature one. Marriage should not take place until the body is healthily and completely developed; to bear offspring prematurely endangers not only the mother's health, but it materially influences the health and well-being of the child.

We cannot fix rigorously the age at which the body becomes fully expanded. I am inclined to say it is at 20 in the female, and at 24 in the male; but original stamina, education, climate, mode of life, etc., have their influence, and may make an earlier or a later marriage proper.

The evil consequences resulting from precocious unions in this country are: diminished vigor and shortened life in the husband; faded beauty, blasted health, and premature old age in the mother, and a diminutive stature, debility of body and imbecility of mind, perhaps a strong predisposition to consumption, rickets, scrofula, etc., in the children.

MARRIAGE SHOULD BE WHEN THE PARTIES ARE IN HEALTH.—I do not say that every ailment should be a bar to marriage or child-bearing. It is possible that prolapsis uteri may be benefited by a pregnancy and parturition. But if a woman has prolapsis uteri, or other ailment, it is a poor preparation for the burdens of gestation, and good health is an important qualification for the responsibilities of married life. No learning can be of more importance to a young lady than to know how to preserve health, and how to restore it when lost, for we cannot reasonably expect healthy children from unhealthy parents. There are numerous other complaints besides scrofula and insanity, inherited by children. If a wife is to be healthy and strong, she must use means; health will not come by wishing for it merely, and whether pleasant at first or not, habit will make early rising, temperate living, taking exercise, thorough ablution of the whole body, etc., easy. That state of vigorous health and strength which prepares a woman to bear strong and vigorous children, is attained not by idleness and luxury, and neglect of personal cleanliness, nor by tight lacing, the use of stimulants, nor by irregular modes of sleeping, etc., but by rising early, and taking early walks in the open air, and engaging in household labor, or other exercise during the day, going to bed betimes, living on an abundance of good, wholesome food, by daily ablutions, followed by rubbing the skin thoroughly, and in general by observing the laws of health. If a woman who has thus preserved her health, marry a man who has been equally careful to observe the laws of continence and hygiene, she may hope to be the mother of a healthy child, and a blessing to all.

THE CONSTITUTION OF BOTH THE MALE AND FEMALE should be good and strong. It is not enough that the body be well developed, if there is at the same time a very feeble constitution. Even if the children of such parents seem to be hale looking and robust, they do not attain old age—are very liable to die young. If there is only a predisposition to disease, such as is often inherited, it may be very doubtful whether the parties ought to marry. If there is only a disposition to habits of intoxication or dissipation, or to gout, madness, scrofula, consumption, etc., in the man, we may advise the woman not to unite herself to him, for these diseases do not show themselves until called into action by some exciting cause.

But we advise the woman, if there is any physical disability which renders her ineligible to the married state, that she should not pass it over lightly, or conceal it, and we would recommend to a woman who may have deformed pelvis, that she abstain from marriage, as she "may purchase the title of wife at too dear a price."

TEMPERAMENT is a matter of less importance in choosing a husband. It is said to be the case that in choosing a mate, a person inclines strongly to one unlike themselves. If it be true that a person of a nervous temperament has a preference for the sympathetic, the sanguine for the bilious, etc., it is probably nature imparts the liking that the offspring may combine the excellence of both, the defects of neither.

BLOOD RELATIONSHIP is not necessarily a bar to union. Cousins may marry when the family has traits of mental and physical excellence as a means of perpetuating them, but it is not best to develop, by repeated unions, a lurking disposition to disease, which may exist in any family.

MORAL AND MENTAL CHARACTER is of the greatest importance. It is not true that "the reformed rake makes the best husband." If he is not the prey of loathsome diseases, the results of a vicious life, his constitution is probably impaired, so that he cannot be the father of good, strong children. The only way that women can guard their own health, and preserve from degeneracy their offspring, is by having husbands of a different character from that of the debauched rake.

CONDUCTOFTHEMOTHERAFTERMARRIAGE.

The mother is accountable for the health and intelligence of her first child; she must be careful of her own health before marriage and at the time of marriage, as well as for the succeeding time.

I will here state a few things which seem unimportant, and yet are of some little consequence. I consider that the great object of conjugal union is the transmission of life, and I cannot believe that anything is unnecessary or unimportant that has a tendency towards the perfect health or well-being of the child that is yet to be born.

DURING THE FIRST FEW MONTHS AFTER MARRIAGE the wife should seek to have bodily quiet, and mental calmness and serenity. The custom of hurrying the bride from place to place may properly be condemned. So we would have her avoid going into a whirl of excitement and pleasure—into a round of visiting and late hours—into close, heated rooms—into fashionable amusements—rich living and a want of rest—sitting in ill-ventilated apartments—quickly bolting unquiet meals—drinking wine, beer, or brandy, or other alcoholic stimulants—late rising in the morning—sleeping in close, badly-ventilated rooms—living in rooms that are kept dark—tight lacing—wearing thin clothing—worrying, and indulging in ill-temper.

She should avoid these at all times, but her future health and happiness depend so much upon her prudence and care during the first year of married life, that we may properly give these hints and cautions in regard to this particular time.

CHAPTER II.
CONDUCT OF THE MOTHER DURING PREGNANCY.

There are no signs of a fruitful conjugation, which in all cases indicate to the woman that she is pregnant. Some few seem to know the exact time; in some instances there is faintness, or vertigo, that in these particular cases impress the fact upon the mind of the woman. But usually, within a month, the point is tolerably certain, she being assured by such signs as will be here pointed out. It now becomes her duty to be especially careful, not only for herself, but also for her offspring. Abortions frequently occur, especially in the first and last pregnancies, and in the first months of pregnancy, these should be avoided if possible.

The train of evils which follow when the habit of abortion is established, as well as the moral obligation she is under to preserve the life committed to her, should make her willing to endure the few privations and conformities which her situation imposes on her. She must avoid undue exercise of the muscles, such as long walks, dancing in hot weather, hastily running up stairs, lifting heavy weights; she must avoid things that inordinately hurry the circulation, such as heated rooms, stimulating liquors, etc.; she must not overload the stomach, or eat late suppers; she must not take drastic purgatives; must not constipate her bowels by taking laudanum, etc.; must not compress the chest by tight lacing; must not use strong tea or narcotics; must not lie long in warm feather beds, and must not engage in severe study, night watching, etc.

The pregnant woman need not indulge in a wayward or voracious appetite, and, although there is a tendency to fullness and fever, she need not necessarily be bled.

The pregnant woman needs fully as much food as usual, but she must avoid excess in eating and drinking. Ripe fruits, lamb, veal, fresh fish, milk, coffee, and, in general, every thing which agrees with the stomach may be eaten; the taste, as a rule, is a safe guide, and may be reasonably indulged. After the sixth month, she may properly eat four or five meals a day.

The best plan of treatment for one to adopt who has longings is not to give way to them, unless the longings be of a harmless, simple nature.

The CLOTHING of the pregnant woman should be suited to the season; but as the vicissitudes of the weather affect her more than they previously did, she should be dressed rather warm. In general, she should wear flannel drawers, especially during advanced pregnancy.

Many women have done themselves an injury by lacing tight to conceal their pregnancy. The dress should be loose and comfortable, nowhere pressing tightly or unequally.

Stays or corsets may be used, in a proper manner, during the first five or six months; they should be moulded to the shape of the changing figure, and must not depress the nipple or the enlarging breasts. The garters ought to be worn slack; tight garters are very injurious, and if the veins are enlarged or varicose, it will be necessary for her to wear an elastic silk stocking.

Moderate exercise in the open air is proper during the period of pregnancy, and walking is a good kind of exercise; but very long walks, and dancing, ought not to be indulged in. Riding in a wagon over rough roads, and railway traveling, are objectionable.

BATHING should be practiced with great care. A warm bath is too relaxing; a tepid bath once a week is beneficial. Sponging the body every morning with lukewarm water may be practiced, and the skin should be quickly dried with a coarse towel. The temperature of the water may be reduced gradually until it is quite cold. A sitz bath may be used every morning, although it is best to sit in it but a few seconds. If it gives a slight shock, it will be immediately followed by an agreeable glow. Put a little warm water with the cold at first.

Ventilation is of the utmost importance. During the day time, the windows in every unoccupied room in the house ought to be thrown open.

Attention should be directed to keeping the atmosphere in the sitting and sleeping rooms of the house fresh. Many poor people sleep in a very small, close bedroom, and breathe an air that is really poisonous. The lady should see also that the house is kept light, that the drains are in good and perfect order; that the privies are frequently emptied of their contents, and that the drinking water supply be not contaminated.

SLEEP, by its sedative influence, and by the calmness of all the functions that attend it, has a favorable influence upon the disturbed nervous system of the mother, and upon the growth of the fœtus. Her bedroom ought to be large and airy, and she should not have curtains closely drawn about her bed. The windows of the room should be opened during the day; the bedclothes should be thrown back, and everything ventilated; the bed must not be loaded with clothes, and the bedroom at night should be dark, and as far as possible from noise. These things will tend to secure sleep; but if the pregnant woman should still be restless, and feeling oppressed and hot, she should perhaps admit more air into the room. Let her also attend every day to her bowels, that they be not allowed to become costive; perhaps eat cooling fruits, live on an abstemious diet, and if there is a feeling of faintness when she attempts to lie down, she should have a bed so arranged that her shoulders and head are elevated.

The pregnant woman ought to retire early to rest, and I would advise her to lie abed in the morning as long as she can sleep well. If she cannot sleep well, let her get up in good time in the morning, take a bath, or thorough ablution, a stroll in the garden, an early breakfast, and then perhaps a short walk, while the air is cool and exhilarating. A nap of an hour or two after that, upon a sofa or lounge, will prove very refreshing.

A TRANQUIL MIND is of the greatest importance. Forebodings of a gloomy nature should not be encouraged, as they often are, by relating dismal stories, etc. Unnecessary fear upon the part of the mother may have a bad effect upon the child, as may also the indulgence in unbridled anger, or yielding to temper,—perhaps may cause convulsions or hemorrhage, or even abortion. There is reason to believe that the imagination of the mother has an influence on the beauty of the child; and it is quite certain that cheerfulness and equanimity of mind contributes to the future good health of the child, and may even affect its disposition and mental traits.

CHAPTER III.
DISEASES OF PREGNANCY .

Pregnancy is not a disease. Many women enjoy better health during its continuance than any other time, and in general the pregnant woman is not quite as much exposed to contagious and other diseases. But there are certain disorders incident to pregnancy, of which it is necessary to speak.

MORNING SICKNESS, when it is only troublesome during the early part of the day, is generally borne without much complaint, or much medical care. Before taking any medicine for it, I advise that the lady try such simple means as the following: Let her take a cup of coffee or milk, and eat a few crackers or a biscuit, after washing her hands and face, and before rising in the morning; then let her remain in bed for about fifteen minutes, then dress quickly and take a short walk. If the sickness continues, let her eat freely of pop corn, and she may eat of this occasionally during the day, or whenever she is suffering from sickness, and let her partake of other food also during the day. Persistent sickness and vomiting indicates a disordered condition of the digestive apparatus, and requires appropriate remedies. Use successively the following: Formula 85, 104, 81, 107.

VOMITING is sometimes so persistent and severe that the stomach can retain nothing, or but very little food. Of course, such cases demand the aid of a physician, and his efforts to give relief may be effectual, when the medicine here directed fails.

COSTIVENESS is another complaint to which pregnant women are liable. This is hurtful in its consequences, being not uncommonly the cause of fever, tenesmus, pain in the bowels, and abortion. Care must be taken to obviate costiveness by the use of such food as will have a laxative effect. The use of graham bread, oatmeal gruel, raisins, figs, grapes, roasted apples, baked pears, brown bread, cracked wheat, stewed prunes, and other varieties of farinaceous food and fruit, may obviate the necessity of taking opening medicines (F. 108, or milk of magnesia.) An enema is an excellent remedy, and every lady should have a good enema apparatus, by which she can administer an injection to herself, and if she suffer from constipation, she should take an enema twice or three times a week, and the early morning is the best time. The clyster may be warm water, or castile soap and water, of the temperature of new milk. It may be well to give occasionally an aperient to insure a thorough clearance of the whole bowels, and castor oil, salad oil, citrate of magnesia, seidlitz powder, stewed rhubarb, or an electuary of figs may be given. I sometimes direct that the woman should take every day a small dose of oil, in a cup of water gruel or oatmeal gruel.

SEVERE PAIN in the bowels and rectum is sometimes caused by a column of hard and indurated feces, which remain for a number of days in the rectum and colon. Not only pain but inflammation, and other serious ills, may result if such a condition is neglected. If taking injections does not suffice to give relief, manual assistance is necessary. The nurse should learn the art of removing them if necessary; she should use a convenient instrument, carefully conducting it into the anus, or she may thrust her finger into the vagina to break the hard mass, and assist in its expulsion, then she should wash it out with repeated clysters.

FOR ABDOMINAL PAINS that are caused by its distention, and by the weight of the enlarged uterus, the woman should wear a bandage, or an abdominal supporter, adjusted to fit the abdomen, and made with proper straps and buckles to accommodate the increasing size of the abdomen. To relieve the pain, the abdominal walls may be rubbed with equal parts of sweet oil and laudanum.

Troublesome HEMORRHOIDS may be caused by constipation, and also by the congestion in the parts, and by the pressure made on the vessels of the part by the enlarged uterus. It is proper sometimes to use emollient fomentations and cataplasms. Relief may often be given by making firm and gentle pressure between the finger and thumb of each distinct tumor, till they are all compressed and returned within the anus.

In cases of BLEEDING PILES, blood comes away each time the patient has a stool. The patient ought to be as quick as possible in relieving the bowels, and should not at such times sit one moment longer than is absolutely necessary. If the piles are inflamed and painful, foment them three times a day, and for half an hour each time, with hot water containing a little carbolic acid—a one per cent. solution. Apply it by means of a sponge. Extract witch hazel may be used also, and relief may often be obtained by sitting over the steam of hot water for fifteen or twenty minutes. Simply put hot water in a close vessel, and sit over it. Sometimes the woman cannot sit in an ordinary chair, and she should sit either on an air cushion, or a water cushion half filled with water, placed on the chair. (F. 107.)

DIARRHŒA is a less frequent attendant of pregnancy than constipation, and the latter is sometimes the cause of the former; in such cases an aperient is required. (F. 109.) Should the complaint remain after the operation of the laxative, opiates are proper, mixed with some mild astringent medicine, aromatics, antacids, etc. (F. 69, 74, 79, 80, 95.)

TENESMUS, and also diarrhœa, are common attendants on abortion, of which they are, indeed, sometimes the cause. Ipecac in half grain doses, with powdered opium, and given every six hours; or frequently repeated doses of opium may be needed. (F. 91, 92.) A flannel bag filled with hot table salt, and applied near the part affected, may give great relief to pain.

HEARTBURN is a common and often a distressing symptom of pregnancy. I would prescribe in such cases an abstemious diet, pepsin, ingluvin, and other medicine to help digestion; antacids and laxatives. (F. 71, 72, 74.) Calcined magnesia is good; prepared chalk is harmful.

It is not necessary for me to dwell upon the few ailments that occasionally afflict pregnant women that I have not yet referred to,—a few words must suffice. If a woman who is pregnant is apt to be FAINT, or to FAINT AWAY, I advise that she be laid down—that she lie flat on her back, with a pillow under her head—that tight articles of dress be loosened—windows raised—water should be sprinkled on her face, a few drops of aromatic ammonia may be administered, and perhaps smelling salts or hartshorn held to the nose. If it is simply fainting, it is not dangerous.

A nervous pregnant woman is sometimes subject to PALPITATION OF THE HEART, especially when lying down. A small dose of aromatic ammonia will generally give relief.

If CRAMPS of the legs or thighs are troublesome, take F. 92, and tie a handkerchief around the limb, above the part affected, and let it remain a few minutes, and use friction. If cramp attacks the bowels or back, a hot bag of salt, or a stone bottle filled with hot water and wrapped in flannel, may be pressed against the part, and something similar should be placed to the sole of the feet.

If PRURITIS PUDENDI—irritation and itching of the external parts—are troublesome, use F. 195, 217, 220, and take frequently a tepid salt and water sitz bath, remaining but a short time in the bath. If the parts are hot and

inflamed, and covered with an eruption, use either of the following lotions:
F. 217, 195.

CHAPTER IV.
INSTRUCTIONS TO A WOMAN DURING THE LAST MONTH OF PREGNANCY.

1. DO NOT TAKE TOO MUCH EXERCISE.—You may get relief from some of your ailments by lying down considerably during the day. If there is leucorrhœa (whites), strangury (a frequent inclination to void the urine), incontinence (an inability to hold the water), pain in the hips with numbness of the inferior (lower) extremities—if the veins of the leg become varicose —if there are anasarcous swellings of the inferior extremities—if there is a pendulous belly, the woman ought not to so exercise as to produce fatigue. She may get some relief by sitting or reclining in the way that is most agreeable.

2. USE MEANS TO HARDEN THE NIPPLES.—Those women who have never had children ought to observe, before labor, whether there is a depressed condition of the nipples; whether they contract as the breasts increase in size. If they do, the condition can be corrected by wearing nipple shields on them. And to harden the nipples: For at least a month before labor, two or three times a day, rub them between the thumb and finger, and bathe them in tincture of myrrh or cologne water, in which a little alum has been dissolved. This will render the skin less sensitive, and avert the distress occasioned by the tenderness of the nipples. If there is especial reason to apprehend excoriated nipples, as there is when they are rough and nodulated like a strawberry or raspberry, make a solution of sulphate of zinc, one grain to the ounce of rosewater, in a wide-mouth bottle, and tilt the bottle upon the nipple, and allow it to remain there for a few minutes, several times every day (F. 198, 217.) It is necessary also to protect the part from the pressure of stays and the friction of the flannel vest. The stays may be removed entirely, or the nipple may be protected by laying a soft linen rag, wet with water and cologne, around it so that the pressure will not be directly on the nipple. If the breasts are swollen or painful, the soreness will subside of itself before the commencement of labor. It may be well,

however, to foment them with flannel wrung out of hot water, and support them as in a sling by a broad handkerchief, passing over the opposite shoulder.

3. PAY NO ATTENTION TO THE CHILLING AND "HORRIFYING TALES OF GOSSIPING BELDAMES."—A cheerful flow of spirits which arises from the hope of a happy event, inspires a woman with activity and resolution, and is the best preparation for the pains of labor. Do not give way to gloomy and melancholy forebodings or indulge in idle reveries. Any person is your enemy who would exaggerate to you the dangers of labor; and let me here say to you, that if you read in this book of certain unfavorable contingencies, do not let your mind dwell upon them; they occur very rarely indeed, and I hope I have given such advice and instruction, and that you have been so cautious and careful that your chance is unusually favorable.

4. DO NOT EXPOSE YOURSELF AT THIS TIME TO WET AND COLD.—Do not go out in bad weather, and do not go to theatres and other crowded places at all. You are especially liable at this time to renal difficulties, and if you take cold, it will cause congestion of the kidneys, and more or less urinary difficulty. It is easier to prevent such complaints than to cure them.

5. TAKE BUT LITTLE MEDICINE.—In general you may rest in the hope that all your troubles will vanish after your confinement, and you can hardly hope to cure them sooner. But keep your bowels loose. If you cannot have daily passages by eating fruits, bread made from unbolted flour, or other laxative diet, take saline waters, compound licorice powder, etc., (F. 108.) If your bowels are constipated at the time that labor commences, take at that time an active cathartic (F. 109).

6. SEEK AND ENGAGE THE BEST POSSIBLE PHYSICIAN.—I do not know but the educated monthly nurse of the future may be well qualified to do all that is necessary in an ordinary natural parturition. But heretofore very few nurses trained in this country are thus prepared; perhaps the popular sentiment is against such an education. But you must always select a physician that you can confide in and trust if an operation is necessary, or there is unusual difficulty.

7. IT IS GENERALLY WELL TO HAVE YOUR PHYSICIAN SEE YOU A MONTH BEFORE THE TIME THAT YOU EXPECT TO BE CONFINED.—Indeed, I would have you consult with your physician during the whole period of your pregnancy. You may get very full directions from this book, but still, where it is practicable, I advise that you consult with some skilled medical friend, who

knows your idiosyncracies, and can suggest modifications of the directions as your own case demands. Specimens of your water should be analyzed each week during the last month, if there are any signs of albuminaria, etc., (especially if the face and ankles are bloated.) If there is inability to pass the water, it may be necessary to draw it with a catheter.

8. SUBMIT YOURSELF ENTIRELY TO THE DIRECTION OF YOUR PHYSICIAN.—Do not indulge in any opinion that may clash with his, even if that opinion is founded upon what is here written; you cannot expect to know more than he. It may be that he will wish to examine you by palpation, etc., to know if the fœtus lies as it should do, as something may be done to correct a malposition by external manipulation if the effort is made early. No good physician will permit that your sensibilities should be shocked by an unreasonable demand. If you have studied this book diligently you will be prepared to converse intelligently with your physician, and you will understand and appreciate any directions that he may give. If you have taken any medicine prepared from formula herein inserted, you know, and can inform him what the medicine is; this is better than it would be if you had taken patent medicine, of the ingredients of which you are ignorant. Consult with your physician in regard to the choice of a nurse, as he will be likely to know those that understand their business, and that are in the habit of following the doctor's directions, or he may know whether the one you selected is now attending a woman that has contagious disease.

9. CHOOSE A GOOD NURSE.—You should have the best possible aid that the nature of circumstances will permit. Do not get a fine lady nurse that requires to be constantly waited on by a servant, and do not get a croaker that discourses of the sad and dreadful cases that have occurred in her experience. Do not get any one that is addicted to intemperance, or a potterer that is devoid of method and efficiency; that does the wrong thing in the wrong way, and that is always out of her proper place. Get a nurse that will not dose and medicate either the mother or child when they are under the care of a physician, or assume any duty or responsibility that belongs to him; that admits that the doctor is the one to give orders. Get one that never reveals the private concerns of her former employers; one that is not a mischief-maker, causing dissention and disagreement in the household. Do not get one that is young, if she is giddy and thoughtless and inexperienced, nor one that is old, if she is deaf and stupid. Get, preferably, a married woman or a widow; one that has at some time had the care of

infants; one that has a pleasant countenance, and is naturally cheerful; one that has calmness and self possession, and firmness, and at the same time is gentle, kind, good-tempered and obliging; she should have a light step, a pleasant voice, a cheering smile, a dextrous hand, a gentle touch, and be gifted in cooking for the sick. By preference, engage a monthly nurse; she will not be so likely to come to you from a case of scarlet fever or erysipelas, or other contagious disease.

If you can find a nurse of the kind described above, and if she be properly instructed and educated, she will be invaluable to you, and if she devotes her talents and her best energies to you and your infant, she should be liberally paid. But there are many such women all over the country, or will be when we can induce them to qualify themselves by study and special effort. But, as really good nurses are full of engagements, it may be necessary for you to engage her in the early months of your pregnancy; only stipulate in the start that you will be obliged to dispense with her services, if it happens that immediately preceding your confinement she had been attending a woman that had puerperal fever.

I do not say that you should necessarily engage a nurse that is educated as a midwife. But such a one is to be preferred even if you have a physician, and then the latter need not be detained from his patients for so long a period of time; and if the last stage of the labor is so rapid that the child is born before the doctor arrives, there need be no trepidation; she will know well what to do. Thousands are born in this country without the slightest assistance from a doctor, he not being at hand nor not being in time, and yet both the mother and babe do well almost invariably. As a rule the nurse that has studied and learned the most is the best prepared to discharge the duties resting upon her.

A NURSE MAY PROPERLY BE IN ATTENDANCE A WEEK OR MORE BEFORE THE TERMINATION OF PREGNANCY, if circumstances permit or require it. If present she will attend to the following things: Choose a good airy room for the lying-in chamber—one that can be well ventilated, where the temperature can be kept at from 60° to 65°; one that is removed as much as possible from noise and disturbance, and where the patient need not be exposed to draughts. Provide needed articles of clothing for mother and child, and dressings for the bed; short gowns to wear over the chemise or ordinary night gown; a proper bandage of heavy muslin, as much as one and a quarter yards in length and fourteen inches in width. I prefer to have it of several thicknesses, and if it is quite long so that the ends meet to be folded it keeps in place better, and if it is gored it should be in such a manner that it is narrower at the lower edge than it is two inches above, so as to prevent it when adjusted from sliding upwards; the child's binder, preferably some woolen material about five inches in width and fourteen inches in length; the child's shirt (woolen or cotton, not starched); both a long and a short petticoat; a frock or slip; a shawl or flannel blanket; napkins and muslin diapers; also pieces of old muslin to be used to absorb blood and water. Provide also for dressing the bed, a piece of impervious oiled cloth, oiled silk, or rubber cloth; old sheets and comfortables; a piece of carpet; have in readiness a pair of shears or scissors, a small box of prepared lard or vaseline or a flask of salad oil, a package of pins one and a half inches in length, besides ordinary pins; tape, bobbin or wrapping twine; fine toilet soap; fine sponge for washing the child; soft linen or carbolated cotton for dressing the naval; a box of unirritating powder; a pile of towels, and a little aromatic ammonia or brandy to be used in an emergency. Let every thing be placed in such order that either may be found without hurry or bustle at a moment's notice. Hot and cold water should always be in readiness.

CHAPTER V.
DIRECTIONST OTHEMONTHL YNURSE.

If you attend a woman to whom the physician has already been called, you will thereafter be subject entirely to his orders. Whatever your opinion is, notwithstanding you have this book or any good authority for your opinion, if it seems to conflict with his directions, obey him; on him rests the responsibility and he is presumed to know what is best. But it is best that you should confide in each other—be on such relations that you can communicate to him anything you have learned about the case; be free to ask of him explicit directions and instructions. But your duties may precede his as well as accompany them, and I wish now to give special directions in regard to things that first demand your attention.

1. A nurse may properly provide a soft rubber catheter and also a syringe; this should be constructed so that it acts as an enema apparatus when one pipe is used, and as a vaginal syringe when the other pipe is applied. The holes in this pipe should be made so that the fluid injected is thrown backward.

It is important that this last direction be observed. I know of one instance where the vaginal pipe of a Davidson syringe was used, yet the fluid injected passed through the cavity of the uterus and through the Fallopian tube and entered the cavity of the peritoneum, causing severe pain and inflammation.

Besides the things already mentioned, I advise that there be furnished for use if needed a small blanket to receive the baby, a little bath tub, two chamber vessels, a bed pan, carbolic acid, fluid extract of ergot, and chloroform.

2. Being employed as a monthly nurse, do not (except very rarely indeed in an emergency) give any medicine at all or any stimulant that has not been ordered by the attending physician. Many women do not consider that labor is a natural process; it is painful indeed, and often lingering and tedious, but will go to a safe termination ordinarily without interference; any medicine given, unless very wisely administered, is much more likely to do harm than good.

3. Be still and noiseless as possible in doing necessary duties when your patient is trying to sleep, or when she is in special need of sleep. Sleep

may be of great importance to her, and it may be put to flight by a little carelessness in renewing the fire, or in walking if you wear heavy and creaking shoes. Nurses at these times should wear slippers and not shoes.

4. If you attend the lady for a week or more before the doctor is called, there may be different ailments which you ought to note, at least enough to know their true significance. Perhaps she has false pains, and suffers so much that she believes that labor has commenced. You will decide partly from the character of the pains. False pains are colicky, though they may shift occasionally from the bowels to the back and loins and may extend to the hips and thighs. They come at irregular intervals, are sometimes violent and sometimes feeble, and they are particularly troublesome at night.

Spurious pains are often caused by disordered stomach and may be somewhat relieved by attention to the diet and by mild aperients (F. 108, 109), or by applying a flannel bag of hot salt. If quite severe send for the doctor; do not give stimulants.

5. You may benefit the patient at this particular time when labor is approaching, perhaps without giving her medicine. Possibly she may feel very well for a day or two, and you will need to direct her exercise so that she does not do too much. You may keep from her unpleasant sights and seeming dangers; keep her room from being overheated; see that she does not have late suppers, too great a quantity of food, or anything that will produce a costive state of the bowels. See that her clothing is not too light, that she does not have strong tea or coffee, and that she does not lie too much in the bed. Secure as much as possible tranquility and equanimity, by guarding against gusts of passion, by keeping from her tales of horror and disaster which have happened to the pregnant, by teaching her that she has nothing to fear in regard to her child from the simple fact that some longing has been ungratified or that she was appalled at some frightful object, as such fears are seldom if ever realized; relieve her if possible of gloomy forebodings by informing her how rarely death happens after a well conducted labor.

6. If you give any medicine at this time give only that which is unirritating and mild.

7. Notice all the indications of approaching labor, the sinking down of the uterus in the pelvis, the contractions of the womb that come on without pain, or with slight pain, the change in the mind and temper of the lady, the augmented mucous secretion, &c.

CHAPTER VI.
CARE OF THE MOTHER DURING LABOR AND CONFINEMENT.

TRUE LABOR PAINS are distinguished from the false by the fact that they are felt considerably in the back, passing down to the thighs, and by their coming on at regular intervals. At first they recur nearly every two hours, and they steadily increase in number and frequency, and are grinding in their character. There are other signs which denote the actual commencement of labor; there is usually a frequent desire to empty the bowels and bladder, perhaps shiverings or rigors unattended with a sensation of cold, sometimes a severe rigor, and these signs are preceded or accompanied or followed by a discharge of mucus and blood, called the show.

It is well now to send for the medical man, though if he lives near by it is only necessary to let him know that his services may shortly be required. If the patient suffers from nausea, vomiting, or chills and shiverings, let her know that they are only incidents of her labor and not unfavorable. Do not let her increase the pains or attempt to increase them in any way; it is much better that the labor should progress in a natural manner, even if it is very slow.

THE PREPARATION OF THE BED for the occupancy of the mother is now to be attended to. Cover the right side of the bed (as the patient will probably lie on her left side) with a piece of water-proof cloth or oil cloth; upon the top of this a sheet is to be placed and fastened with safety pins. Over this permanent dressing (on the top of the bed sheet) a neatly folded draw sheet is adjusted (and a second rubber and draw sheet is desirable), which, after the labor, can be removed, leaving the first clean and dry. This second draw sheet and rubber, and also a folded comfortable can be placed a little nearer the foot of the bed than the other, and after the lady's confinement she can be drawn up on the permanent dressing, and the temporary dressing can be easily removed. The other bedclothes may be adjusted in the usual manner.

A piece of carpet can be thrown on the floor by the side of the bed, and it is well to have a hassock to put between the patient's feet and the foot-board or bed-post.

To dress for the occasion, a folded sheet should be adjusted around the waist (or, instead of this, or above this, a petticoat), to extend from the waist to the feet. (These will be removed after the delivery.) Then a chemise should be put on in the usual manner, and drawn up and folded high under the arms. She should then have on a clean nightgown, and over it a warm wrapper; this can easily be slipped off when she is about to go to bed, and the night-dress, if it is a long one, can be folded up under her arms, so that it will not be soiled.

The stays must not be worn, as that prevents the free action of the muscles of the chest and abdomen. The patient, during the first stage of labor, may walk about or sit down, and need not confine herself to the bed. She may be allowed such food as she can eat, but should not be urged to take food.

The best beverage for her is either a cup of warm tea, or of gruel or arrowroot. Cold water will not hurt her if she desires it. A patient ought, during labor, frequently to pass water. Some women, from false delicacy, do not attend to it, and suffer severely for it.

The doctor ought to have some room to retire to that the patient may be left very much to herself, and that she may have opportunity whenever she desires to of thoroughly emptying either the bladder or bowels. It is better that not more than two women be present with her, and even one of these can be dispensed with if necessary.

The room should be kept quiet.—Let the attendants be quiet and self-possessed, and let there be no noise, or excitement, or whispering. There may be ordinary cheerful conversation, but when the pains become very frequent and severe, it is best that this should be hushed enough to have the patient feel that the attendants are not neglectful of her, or careless about her. Cheerful words spoken to the patient of the blessed relief that will come after enduring so much pain will do good.

When the membranes are ruptured and the waters discharged, the doctor should be called in immediately. When he is present you will be subject entirely to his direction.

If the medical man cannot be present pretty soon, I advise any nurse who has diligently studied this book to make a digital examination, and ascertain if there is a head presentation; if there is, there need not be any anxiety about getting a doctor.

If the child is born before the doctor has time to reach the house, let the patient be made to understand that there is not the slightest danger; and, for yourself, observe the following directions:

Ascertain if a coil of naval string be about the neck of the infant; if there is, remove it immediately. See that it has room to breathe; that there is not a membrane over its mouth, and that its face is not buried in the clothes or the discharges. If the child cries, give a minute's attention to the mother, to see that she is in an easy position, and for a few minutes make pressure with one hand over her abdomen. If the child does not cry the moment it is born, give it a smart blow on the back, sprinkle a little cold water upon it, and put your finger in its mouth to remove any mucus that may interfere with respiration.

After the child cries, and when no pulsation can be felt in the cord, tie and cut it. Tie with a strong and not too fine a string, about one and a half inches from the child's body, and cut so as to leave that portion of the cord attached to the child's body about two and a half inches long. Cut far enough from the ligature so that it will not be liable to slip off. The ligature should be drawn tight when applied, and it ought to be examined afterwards to know that it does not continue to bleed.

I shall here summarize, in a very brief way, what you are to do in the absence of the doctor: After the child is breathing properly and the cord is cut, the mother may receive your attention. If the placenta is not expelled spontaneously, place one or both your hands over the uterus, and by friction, squeezing and pressure there, you will probably cause enough contraction of the womb to start the placenta from its attachments. You may then make slight traction on the cord, pulling only gently, and it will probably come down; as it emerges from the vagina gently twist or turn over the afterbirth, and you will secure the removal of the membranes.

The soiled articles are now to be removed, a binder applied, the patient placed nicely in bed and kept quiet; no talking, no visiting, no excitement allowed.

The baby may now be attended to—be washed and dressed. Have at hand a bowl of warm water, a small quantity of lard or oil, soap, fine sponge, and the articles of clothing, including a binder, and by preference a piece of flannel for washing. It is well also to have a small tub large enough to dip the child in. If the child is much covered with the "vernix caseosa," rub it over with some unctuous substance, and then wipe it off with the flannel or some soft cloth, being careful at the same time that nothing gets into the eyes of the child, and being careful to remove all the cheesy matter from the angles of the joints, and from behind the ears. Have the water for the bath warm, but not hot; take hold of the feet of the child with your right hand and putting the left under its back and shoulders, lower it into the water, supporting its head by your arm. While supporting its head with your left hand, wash it all over, using toilet soap and (if you have it) a fine, clean sponge; then lift it out into a warm towel and dry it thoroughly. Dust with fine starch powder, made of wheaten flour, under the arms and between the legs, and dress the naval by using a soft piece of linen dipped in vaseline and having a hole in the center. It is well to put another piece of linen around the cord, which may then be turned upward or to the left side, and the binder applied. Some prefer to put absorbant cotton around the cord. The binder or belly-band should be made of flannel, and should be cut bias. Care should be taken to apply it tight enough not to slip, but too tight an application should be particularly avoided. All the garments of the child should be made subservient to comfort and not to show; should be warm and not too small; should consist in part of flannel during cool weather. When dressing the child put one garment inside the other, and put the whole on over the feet. But few pins need to be used if the clothes be properly arranged; three pins are sufficient for the binder. The washing or dressing of the child should be done quickly; a little cold water should be given it; it should be all the time in a warm room, and may be laid where it is quite warm.

The mother may demand a little more attention before the child is applied to the breast. A folded napkin should at first have been applied to the vulva. Look to it and see if it is much soiled with blood. When it is, apply a clean one, and observe particularly that one is placed so that it is partly under her; observe if her bandage is well retained in its place, and if it presses well on the lower portion of the bowels. If the binder is kept well adjusted it does good; it is of no use if it is allowed to slip up from its place. A towel folded and laid over the lower portion of the bowels, under the bandage, is useful as a compress, and helps to keep the binder in place.

Everything should be arranged so that the patient can have rest and quietness; but before she goes to sleep put the child to the breast. If the nipple is retracted, an ordinary tobacco pipe may be used to draw it out so that the child can get hold of it. If the child draws on the breast, the milk which it obtains will serve to physic it, and it should be applied to the breast every four or five hours; nothing else need be given it, except perhaps a little sugar and water.

If necessary to induce the child to take the breast, a little sweetened water or sweetened milk may be applied to the nipple. While the child is nursing the mother may lay upon her side, and receive the child upon the arm of that side upon which she is lying. Perhaps, in order to draw out the nipple so that the child can grasp it in its mouth, it may be necessary to use some bottle with a flat, smooth mouth; fill the bottle with hot water; after a minute, empty it and place the mouth of the bottle immediately over the nipple; as the bottle cools there will be sufficient suction to elevate the sunken nipple.

Soon after the termination of the labor the woman may partake of some light food—tea and toast, panada, or anything of a light, unirritating character. From the very first, under ordinary circumstances, the woman may be permitted to change her position as she may desire, from side to side, or to be propped up in bed. Before going to sleep she ought to urinate —in a lying position, if so inclined, or she can be raised up and supported in a sitting position for a few minutes, if she desires to be. The patient must not be allowed to exert herself, or remain too long in a sitting posture. But I have never known a woman to be harmed by being raised up and sitting for a minute at this particular time.

Unless there is unusual suffering from afterpains or hemorrhage, or something that requires the attention of the physician, the patient will now be desiring and seeking sleep, and everything should be arranged for this object.

CHAPTER VII.
DIRECTIONS TO THE NURSE DURING THE MONTH.

The nurse will receive from the medical man such directions as the peculiarities of the case seem to demand, but I deem it proper here to give some general instructions. First, in regard to

CARE OF THE MOTHER.

REST is essential to the mother during the month. She should remain in bed nearly all the time for at least two weeks, and should not return to her household duties under a month. Perfect tranquility is essential, that the womb may resume its former size and situation, and that inflammation, ulceration, prolonged debility, pain and excessive discharges be avoided, and that a good form be preserved. As a means of preventing a flabby, pendulous belly, she may also, when she does walk around, wear a utero-abdominal supporter or a well-fitting bandage. If a bandage is worn it should be made of strong linen, cut bias, setting snugly to the form, but not exerting unpleasant pressure. Its breadth should be from twelve to eighteen inches.

The diet of a nursing woman should be both light and nourishing. I would suggest for the first day well-boiled gruel, bread and milk, panada, tea, dry toast and butter, or bread and butter. For the second day, beef tea may be added (F. 58), and she should be served with food four times; the third day she may eat a little chicken or game, and mashed potatoes or rice pudding, and on the fourth day she can partake once of mutton or beef. Arrow root (F. 44), with these articles mentioned, may form part of her diet thereafter, but she may partake of such articles of her former diet as are wholesome and nourishing. The woman must not be starved; she demands food that will allow her to recuperate her strength. Give her as nutritious food as she has appetite for, and can easily digest and assimilate. (F. 58.)

For a BEVERAGE give toast water, barley water, and milk with the chill taken off and a little salt added, tea, cocoa, or chocolate made with one-half milk, new milk and water, cacao and broma, made with a large proportion of milk. Either of these may be freely used as a drink. I have always allowed my patients to drink freely of water from the first, and an occasional cup of coffee is not harmful. When the mother experiences any inconvenience from any articles of diet or drink, she should not hesitate to abandon them, for if they disagree with her they will also disagree with the child. (F. 10, 16, 18, 19, 20, 23, 25, 28.)

The LOCHIAL DISCHARGE, which occurs directly after a lying-in, is at first of a reddish color, and gradually changes to a brownish hue, and afterwards to a greenish shade. It is necessary that there should be some discharge to continue for a week, and it often continues for three weeks more. In some cases it has a disagreeable odor.

ABLUTIONS and cleansings are very necessary at this time. The parts should be carefully cleansed every day, and it is never amiss to use for this purpose a weak solution of chlorinated soda, or carbolic acid, or permangenate of potassa, etc., (F. 153.) They may be used quite weak at first, and afterwards of greater strength, if they do not cause smarting. Tar water is excellent for an injection. The woman should daily assume a position that will facilitate the discharge of the lochia; sometimes get on her knees, or she may occasionally lie on her face and stomach. There should be no bandages applied so as to confine the secretions. A soft sponge and warm water may be used for ablutions at first, or the parts may be bathed with warm water and oat meal gruel; after bathing they should be dried with warm, dry towels; they may then, by means of a piece of linen rag, be anointed with salad oil or vaseline, or other bland oil. Once or twice a day the vagina should be syringed out with some injection. (F. 153, 155.)

To WASH OR CLEANSE the patient so that the pores of the skin in every part are free and unobstructed, a soft napkin wet with warm soap and water, should be passed underneath the bedclothing, and she should be rubbed all over without any exposure to a draught of air. In some way she should take a sponge bath every day.

The CLOTHING which a patient will wear immediately after a labor has been already, indicated. As some garments worn during labor are not necessarily soiled, they may be worn until the third or fourth day, when the dress should be changed. This may be done without tiring or exposing the patient. Without raising her up you can pull the bedgown down from over each arm, and after removing it from under the body, you can draw down the chemise and remove it from below. You can place her arms in the sleeves of the clean chemise, throw it over her head and pull it down; and put on a clean bedgown in a similar manner, or both may be put on at once.

The BED CLOTHING as well as the body linen should be changed frequently. In changing the upper sheet it should be pulled off from below, and the clean one can be carried down in its place without removing the other bedclothes, by plaiting the lower half of it. To put on a clean under-sheet, plait one side of it, and place that under the patient while she lies on her side, then let her turn on her back or other side onto it, and draw out the plaited part. Care of this kind is necessary until she is able to sit. Have the sheets well aired, and have a proper temperature in the room.

THE LYING-IN ROOM should always be kept well ventilated and rather cool; it is injurious to the patient to have the room kept at a high temperature. Perhaps the ventilation can be secured by having a little fire in the room, and by occasionally leaving the door of the apartment ajar, at the same time being careful to guard against draughts. But visitors remaining in the room, or any additional number of persons, serve to vitiate the air, as well as to prevent the necessary repose of the patient. A sensation of chilliness may be felt by the woman after delivery, and her feet may be cold; if they are, something warm should be applied to them, and sufficient clothing should be on the bed; but afterwards be careful not to overload her with clothes, as well as to avoid having the room overheated.

TOO MUCH LIGHT in the room may be injurious to the eyes of the mother or child, and it is often necessary to darken the room somewhat for a few days.

The lying-in woman will usually be confined to her room for two weeks. After the first fifteen days she may very properly remove to another room adjoining, or near at hand, and during her absence her room and bed may be ventilated by throwing the windows wide open and throwing the bedclothes back. Ordinarily she may, at the end of three weeks, take her meals with the family, but she ought still to lie down occasionally to rest her back. At about this time she may take an airing in a carriage, if the weather be fine.

All lying-in women ought not to be treated alike in regard to DIET, etc. While a light, unstimulating diet is best at first in ordinary cases, the weak and delicate require good, nourishing food from the commencement, such as beef tea, chicken broth, mutton chops, eggs, etc., (F. 57, 58, 59.) Oatmeal gruel increases the secretion of milk, is nourishing and easily digested, at the same time it is simple and bland, and proper for those that are corpulent, or strong and robust, and the same may be said of good cow's milk. But, as the healthy mother furnishes daily from a quart to a quart and a half, she needs some meat to keep up her strength. Never give stimulants to increase the woman's strength, or to increase the quantity of milk.

In some cases, after a severe and lingering labor, there is RETENTION OF URINE. If the bladder cannot otherwise be emptied, the catheter must be used every six or eight hours.

The bowels are usually costive after a confinement, and I prefer to give a dose of castor oil the third day. If this or some other aperient is not given, enemas should be administered sufficient to cause evacuations.

The care of the MOTHER'S BREASTS is important. Before the milk is abundantly secreted, she should not be fretted by very frequent ineffectual attempts at nursing, though it may be necessary to draw out the nipple by means of a breast pump. The milk should be drawn out when the breasts become full and distended, and they should not be allowed to remain hard and sore. Apply fomentations; cabbage leaves, wilted in hot vinegar and water, or warm solution of carbolic acid, one part to eighty. If they continue to be swelled and painful use F. 221, 223. It may be necessary to make gentle pressure upon them by means of strips of adhesive plaster, or by a sort of jacket or bandage, that should be prepared especially for the purpose. When the breasts are closely bandaged they should be supported on each side by pads of cotton, so that the pressure will be made equally upon them.

Delay in applying the child to the breasts is often a cause of swelled breasts. After it has been fed for a few days it may refuse to nurse, and if it does nurse the nipple may be quite tender. But, unless for some cause the secretion is to be checked, the effort should be made every two hours to induce the child to draw. You will be more successful in these efforts if you can reduce the heat and swelling. Rub the breasts every four hours with good, warm olive oil, vaseline, or camphorated oil, and keep the excoriated nipple thickly coated with sub-nitrate of bismuth.

The breast should be rubbed, and the child should be nursed regularly, although I do not advise that the child or the mother should be roused from their slumbers; it is better to delay for awhile the usual effort. But, even at first, a child can be nursed with considerable regularity every hour and a half during the day, and twice during the night; and it should be applied alternately to either breast, even if it seems to prefer one to the other.

It is often necessary to wash the breast and nipple with warm water, and dry it with a soft napkin, before applying the babe.

During all the time that the mother nurses the child, the MIND OF THE MOTHER exerts an influence on the latter through her milk. If the mother's mind is very much disturbed by any apprehensions, fears or anxieties, these perturbations will not only be likely to check the flow of milk, but will alter its quality, and perhaps render it hurtful and dangerous to the infant. The nurse should guard the patient as much as possible from anything causing nervous agitation, fretting, anger, grief, fear, sudden terror, or great anxiety, as these are injurious to the mother, and may be harmful and fatal to the child. Equanimity and cheerfulness of mind on the part of the mother are important at any period of her pregnancy or nursing. I will now give more particular directions in regard to

THE CARE OF THE CHILD.

THE FOOD OF THE CHILD, if it is necessary to feed it at first, may be one-third of new milk and two-thirds of warm water, slightly sweetened. It is not necessary that it should be fed for at least eight hours after birth, and at first the quantity fed it must be small. Except in rare cases the milk furnished by the mother will come soon enough, and in sufficient quantity to supply the wants of the child, and it is best for both that the child should draw it when secreted. For the instruction of the mother, as well as the nurse, I here quote a paragraph upon the nourishment and feeding of the child, not only of the new-born, but also of the subsequent months:

"No form of artificial nourishment can compare with that furnished by the mother. Women should know and consider the probability of disease and death occurring from any other mode, and the difficulties and annoyances to be encountered in the use of artificial food. As a further inducement to her to nurse her own child, she should know that her offspring is sure to imbibe with its milk, deep, earnest affection. The mother who can nurse her own offspring should commence within eight hours after delivery, and in the mean time no trash should be put in its mouth to still its cries, or for any other reason; if it has not been surfeited, it will be disposed to take the breast. It should be placed to the breast before they are gorged with milk, for at that later time the flow is less easy, the parts are more irritable, and the child sucking with greater power, we are more likely to have, as the result, irritated nipples. Nature prompts all animals to suck their mother soon after they are born; we are less liable to have sore, irritated, cracked nipples, and there is less liability to infantile colics, etc., if we follow the guidance of nature and instinct."

As soon as possible accustom the child to the habit of nursing every two hours. If there is a proper interval between the times of nursing, the child draws with more avidity, actually empties the breast, and obtains that part that contains the most cream. Endeavor also to have the intervals longer at night, so that, from 10 P. M. to 6 A. M., it nurses but once or twice. Still, if it wakes every two or three hours, demands its supply of nourishment, and you cannot otherwise quiet the child, you must indulge it. Do not accustom the child to sleeping on the mother's breast. If it sleep in its own crib or bed, properly clothed and protected, it is less liable to have its rest disturbed. Avoid the custom of having a young child sleep with old and sickly persons, and also of having them sleep in ill-ventilated rooms, and of covering the child's face as it sleeps. There is danger that a child may die from want of pure fresh air, from having its face pressed tightly in the embrace of the person with whom it sleeps, from the multiplicity of its clothes, and from the mass of bedclothing used by the mother, as well as from improper food. A child should never be covered to sweat by reason of the warmth of its clothing, or of that of the apartment.

If the mother does not enjoy good health, it may be better for her not to nurse the child at night, but to have it fed once or twice with a little diluted cow's milk at night, and to nurse it during the day.

The following have been named as CAUSES WHY THE MOTHER CANNOT PROPERLY NURSE THE CHILD:

1. When she cannot have a sufficient quantity of milk.

2. When the supply falls off from some defect which is not remediable.

3. When there is a strong venereal or scrofulous taint in the constitution.

4. When suckling produces an active or painful disease in the mother, as colic, etc.

5. When the mother is subject to great nervous debility; possesses an irascible temperament, and cannot avoid grief and sorrow; and also when she is suffering from certain hereditary chronic diseases.

WHEN A MOTHER CANNOT SUCKLE HER CHILD, if circumstances will allow, a healthy wet-nurse should be procured. Choose one that is of a healthy family; ascertain that there are no eruptions on her skin, or if there be other disease; if she have a plentiful breast of milk, and if it be of a good quality; if she has good nipples, and if her child is born near the time that the one was that she is to nurse. Do not get a nurse that menstruates during suckling, nor one that has a child which is unhealthy, or has a sore mouth or blotches upon the skin.

Very feeble new-born babes cannot take the breast sometimes. In such cases cow's milk, water and sugar (F. 1) may be given in small quantities at a time, but frequently repeated. If it takes only a teaspoonful at a time it should be repeated every half hour.

Many mothers are unable to obtain the services of a wet-nurse. The milk of a cow is the best substitute, and when this is of ordinary richness, it may be diluted with an equal quantity of water, or thin barley water.

The following are leading principles to guide in giving infant food:

1. Aliment should always be presented to the infant stomach in a fluid form.

2. Bread and other farinaceous substances are generally indigestible in the infant stomach, and may better be excluded from infant feeding.

3. Cow's or goat's milk, when pure and modified so as to resemble as much as possible human milk, will generally be found sufficient without any other help to nourish the new-born infant.

4. If cow's milk is used at first, diluted with twice as much water and slightly sweetened, the proportion of water must be gradually lessened, until after six months the milk may be given undiluted.

5. When good milk from one cow cannot be obtained, and the child does not thrive upon the milk used, condensed milk may properly be substituted.

6. There are various forms of infant food referred to in F. 1, 2, 3, 4, 11, 28, 45, 49, and if one of these is tried and proves satisfactory, it will not be advisable to try new kinds of infant food which are at the present time offered for sale. Milk should be the basis of all infantile food; neither starch, dextrine or glucose sufficiently nourishes without it; but we may use one of these foods without milk for one or two days, in unsettled state of the stomach, with good results. (F. 61.)

THOROUGHLY WASH THE BABE EVERY MORNING from head to foot, using a large wash bowl or nursing basin, half filled with water. First wet the head, then immediately put the body in the bath, and with a sponge or piece of flannel, cleanse the whole body, particularly the armpits, groins, and between the thighs. The skin, after being thus cleansed, must be quickly and thoroughly dried with soft towels, and the parts liable to become sore, powdered; then all parts of the body and limbs should be gently rubbed.

During all the time, when the child is but a few days old, it should not be exposed at all to the cold. The water for its bath should be slightly warmer than new milk, and the time occupied in the bathing should be short. Each time, after a passage from the bowels, the parts should be washed with warm water, and if there is any chafing the calamine powder should be applied.

THE NAVAL STRING should receive the attention of the nurse; within an hour of the time it is at first tied, she should examine the dressing to see if there has been any bleeding. If it bleeds, and the doctor is not at hand, retie with a stout cord, drawing it quite tight. Each morning, when the child is bathed, lift up the naval string with the rag dressing and insert a little nice fresh tallow under it. When it is loose remove it, but use no means to cause the separation. The naval is sometimes a little sore, but seldom needs any dressing more than simply vaseline or tallow.

AT NIGHT a child should be entirely undressed, and its clothing replaced by other garments, those that are loose, light, and sufficiently warm for it while it is under the bedclothes. For a very young child the proper night-dress is a loose slip; when older, a pair of drawers, fitting up well around the neck and covering the body and limbs, is a good article. The clothing worn during the day should not be worn at night, and the clothing when soiled should be immediately changed. Whenever the child seems disposed to sleep, this should be encouraged. Never arouse a child suddenly from its sleep. Be careful that there is no unnecessary noises to disturb its sleeping. Time the bathing and dressing so that the little one may not be unnecessarily disturbed. But never give soothing syrups, anodynes for infants, or other nostrums to induce them to sleep. If the child is restless, endeavor to ascertain if there is not some cause that can be removed, such as tight clothing, etc.

PREMATURE INFANTS may, under favorable circumstances and assiduous care, live and thrive. Immediately after birth the child should be placed in a warm bath, and then wrapped in cotton. The baths should be warmer than usual, and must be frequently repeated. Awaken the child every one or two hours to feed it. Milk (woman's milk is the best) must be given it by a teaspoon. With a view to the better development of the lungs, it may be excited to cry by a slight irritation. Do not bring such children into the open air for several months after the birth, as their passages are readily affected.

CHAPTER I.
OF THE PELVIS.

The formative organs of generation are situated within a large cavity, called the cavity of the pelvis, the walls of which are composed of bones and soft parts. This basin (in Latin, *pelvis*) is an irregular, long cavity, situated at the base of the spinal column, and above the inferior extremities. In the adult the bony pelvis may be divided into four parts or bones, viz: the os sacrum, two ossa innominata, and the os coccygis, but in early life they are more minutely divisible.

THE SACRUM.

The sacrum (Fig. 1) terminates the vertebral column, and is perhaps the most important bone in the pelvis, obstetrically considered, as it enters largely into the various deformities of the pelvis. In the adult it is of a triangular shape, the base of the triangle being above and inclining forwards, the apex below and somewhat backwards; its length is from four to four and a half inches; its breadth about four inches, and the greatest thickness, two and a half inches. The internal surface is concave to the amount of half an inch, crossed by four transverse lines, marking the former division by cartilage; here are four pair of holes, through which pass numerous nervous filaments, which afterwards form part of the great sciatic nerve.

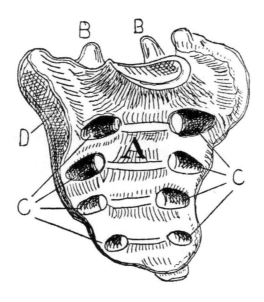

Fig. 1– A   represents the internal or anterior surface of the sacrum.

          B B   represents the articular processes.

          C C   represents the anterior sacral foramen.

          D   represents the articulating surface.

It is placed at the posterior part of the pelvis, where it appears like a wedge forced in between the ossa innominata, immediately below the vertebral column and directly above the coccyx.

THE OSSA INNOMINATA.

The os innominata (nameless bone, Fig. 2) is of a very irregular figure, and the pair occupy the lateral and anterior parts of the pelvis. The external or femoral surface is turned backwards and downwards, as well as outward; at its superior part, inferiorly it looks downwards. Towards the front, the external face presents the cotyloid cavity, or the acetabulum; a little more in advance and below is the subpubic or obturator foramen, which is nearly closed by the obturator ligament.

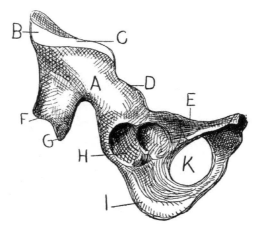

Fig. 2. Right os innominatum, external surface.

Fig. 2—Represents the external surface of the right os innominatum. A. The external iliac fossa; B, crest of the ilium; C, anterior superior spine of the ilium; D, anterior inferior spine of the ilium; E, horizontal branch of the pubis; F, posterior superior spine of the ilium; G, posterior inferior spine of the ilium; H, acetabulum; I, ischium; K, obturator foramen. At birth the haunch bone, or os innominata, is composed of three bones connected by cartilage. Fig. 3.

The superior portion of the bone is characterized on its abdominal or internal face by a large excavation called the internal iliac fossa (Fig. 4.) This portion is terminated below by a large rounded and concave line. The inferior (lower) portion presents behind a nearly triangular plane surface; near the middle of this is the obturator foramen, and in front is the internal face of the os pubis.

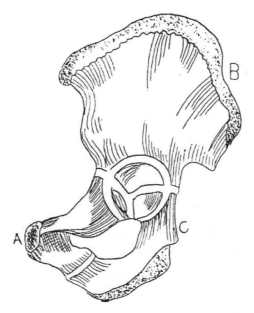

Fig. 3. Left os innominatum, external
surface, etc.

Fig. 3—Left os innominatum, partly
ossified. The haunch bone as it exists in
the child. A, pubis; B, ilium; C, ischium.

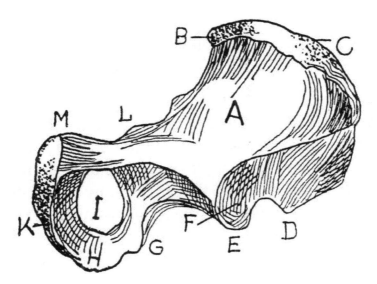

Fig. 4. Right os innominatum, internal surface.

Fig. 4—Right os innominatum, internal surface. A, internal
iliac fossa; B, anterior superior spinous process of the ilium;
C, crest of the ilium; D, posterior superior spinous process
of the ilium; E, posterior inferior spinous process of the
ilium; F, articular surface; G, spine of the ischium; H,
tuberosity of the ischium; I, obturator foramen; K, ischia

pubic ramus; L, crest of the pubis; M, the pectineal eminence.

THE OS COCCYGIS.

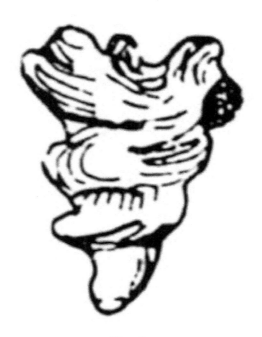

Fig. 5.

The os coccygis.

The OS COCCYGIS (Fig. 5) is three or four little bones united together on the median line of the body, and attached to the os sacrum. Each little bone is tipped with cartilage, and they are so united as to be movable. The entire bones form a pyramid, the apex of which is below. The internal surface is smooth, like that of the sacrum, terminating the plane of the sacrum and bounding it anteriorly.

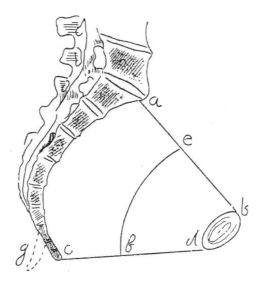

Fig. 6. Vertical section of the pelvis.

Fig. 6—Inlet, outlet, and axis of the pelvis. a, b, plan of inlet—superior strait; c, d, plan of outlet, or inferior strait; e, f, axis of cavity; g, the coccyx extended as it is in labor.

Of the JOINTS OF THE PELVIS it is only necessary here to say that there is no motion in them to facilitate labor, except that the sacro-coccygeal joint is of the kind called ginglymoid, admitting of extensive motion, especially backward, so as to permit the enlargement of the lower outlet an inch or more. (Fig. 6.)

OF THE PELVIS IN GENERAL.

We will now consider the pelvis collectively or as a whole; its relation to the rest of the body; its magnitude, axis, etc. It is connected with the trunk by the articulation of the sacrum with the last lumber vertebra, effected in the same manner as the junction of the vertebra with each other; with the lower extremities it is connected by means of the hip joints. When the pelvis is *in situ*, the brim is neither horizontal nor perpendicular. It represents a cone, slightly flattened from before backwards, the base of which being above, while the apex is directed downwards.

When the body is erect the upper part of the sacrum and the acetabula are nearly on the same descending line, the point of the os coccygis being a little above the arch of the pubis, and the sacro-vertebral angle three inches and nine lines higher than the pubis. Were it not for the obliquity owing to the upright position of the human female, the womb would gravitate low in the pelvis, and produce most injurious pressure on the contained viscera. The lower or true pelvis is the part involved in parturition, and its size and shape demands our attention.

THE BRIM OF THE PELVIS.

This is defined by the LINEO ILIO PECTINEA, which marks the boundary of the true and false pelvis, and this *superior strait* is the entrance of the lesser pelvis. Its form has been variously described as being oval, heart-shaped, and triangular. If we call it "triangular with angles rounded off," the base of the triangle is behind and the apex in front. It would be nearly oval were not the oval form broken by the promontory of the sacrum. This brim is the first solid resistance the head of the fœtus meets in its descent through the pelvis.

DIAMETER OF THE PELVIS.

Different estimates are made by different anatomists of the measurements of the brim of the pelvis. The following is nearly the correct size of the ordinary female pelvis:

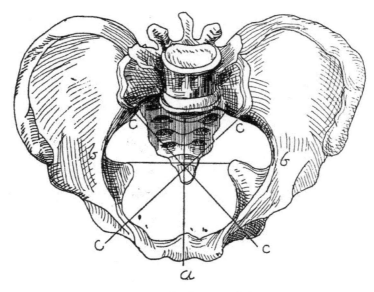

Fig. 7. The bony pelvis.

Fig. 7—The pelvis seen from above. a a, The antero-posterior or sacro-pubic diameter; b b, the transverse diameter; c c, the two oblique diameters.

The circumference varies from thirteen to fifteen inches; the antero-posterior diameter, *i. e.*, from the prominence of the sacrum to the upper edge of the symphasis pubis, (Fig. 6), is about four and a quarter inches; the transverse across the widest part of the brim, at right angles to the antero-posterior, is five and a quarter inches, and the oblique from the sacro-iliac synchondrosis of one side to the opposite of the brim, just above the acetabulum, is five inches. (Fig. 7).

THE CAVITY OF THE PELVIS, of which the fixed boundaries are the sacrum and the pubis, is of unequal depth. The height in front is one and a half inches; upon the sides, three and three-quarter inches, and it is four and a quarter inches if a straight line be drawn from the sacro-vertebral angle to the point of the coccyx, five and a quarter inches following the curve of the sacrum, and six inches if the coccyx be extended. (Fig. 6).

The antero-posterior diameter of the outlet from the arch of the pubis to the point of the coccyx is usually four and a quarter inches, but may increase to five inches during labor by the retrocession of the coccyx (Fig. 8); the transverse from one tuber ischii to another is four and a quarter inches, and the oblique about four and three-quarter inches.

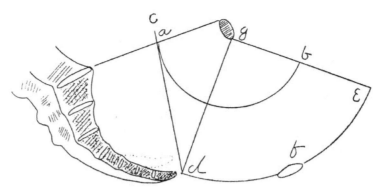

Fig. 8—Position of the pelvis and the axis at the termination of labor.

Fig. 8—a b, Total axis of the excavation; c, the axis of the superior strait; d e, perineum as distended at the moment of the passage of the head.

It is important to notice that the diameters are entirely changed between the rim and the outlet, and that the change is effected gradually. The axes of the inlet and outlet form an obtuse angle with each other (this is illustrated in Figs. 6 and 8.) The three diameters taken at the center of the pelvis are very nearly equal—about four and three-quarter inches.

DIFFERENCES OF THE PELVES.

There is considerable difference between the male and female pelvis, in shape and size. The pelvis in the male is smaller but deeper; the bones are thicker and the brim is more circular, the depth of the symphasis pubis is greater, the sacrum is more perpendicular, the arch of the pubis is narrower, the tuber ischii are nearer each other, and the coccyx less movable. In the female the iliac fossæ are larger, the interval separating the angle of the pubis from the acetabulum is greater, causing the prominence of the hips and wider separation of the thighs, the superior straight is larger and more elliptical, the curve of the sacrum deeper and more regular, the tuberosities of the ischii are further apart, and the arch of the pubis broader. From the greater width of the female pelvis, and from the upper end of the thigh bones being farther apart than in the male, the thigh bones approach each other in their descent, giving a peculiarity to the movements of the female in walking.

The soft parts lining the pelvis and covering it externally modify the diameters of the pelvis, but the effect of these additions in diminishing the internal diameter is not very great. The diameter of the cavity is lessened thereby from one-fourth to one-half an inch.

USES OF THE PELVIS.

One function of the pelvis is to inclose and protect the bladder, rectum and seminal vesicles of the male, the uterus, Fallopian tubes and ovaries, as well as the bladder and rectum in the female. During labor it affords a passage for the child.

TERMINAL OUTLET OF THE PELVIC CANAL.

This is not at the coccyx, but rather at the anterior commissure of the perineum. This is so greatly distended at the last moment of labor as to much prolong the posterior wall of the pelvic excavation and the canal to be traversed by the fœtus. (Fig. 8).

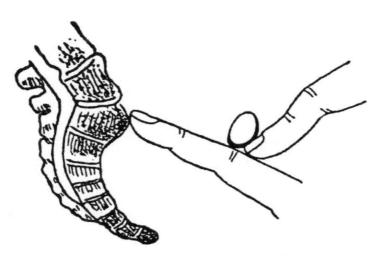

Fig. 9—Section of sacrum and pubis.

Measuring superior strait.

CHAPTER II.
PARTS CONTAINED IN THE PELVIS.

The internal organs of generation are the vagina and uterus with its appendages; but I will first describe the urethra and the perineum.

The URETHRA is a membranous dilatable canal about an inch and a half in length, and directed obliquely from before backwards, and from below upwards, running under and behind the symphasis pubis, from which it is separated by loose celular tissue. Its inferior portion is intimately united to the vaginal walls. Its meatus, the outlet for the urine, is situated about an inch from the clitoris, and immediately above the prominent enlargement of the anterior part of the vagina.

Internally the urethra opens into the bladder. Its direction is subject to variation during pregnancy, the bladder being carried upwards with the uterus, the urethra curves under the pubic arch, and then ascends perpendicularly. The same change occurs when the uterus is enlarged from other causes. In prolapse of the pelvic viscera the course is reversed.

The PERINEUM is the portion between the rectum and the vagina.

THE UTERUS.

The uterus is the organ provided for the reception, growth, and ultimately for the expulsion of the fœtus. In the virgin normal state it is pear-shaped, flattened from before backwards; is situated in the cavity of the pelvis, between the bladder and the rectum, and projects into the upper end of the vagina below. Its upper end or base is directed upwards and forwards, so that its axis corresponds very nearly with that of the superior strait, and forms an angle with the vagina.

The uterus measures about three inches in length, at its upper part two in breadth, an inch in thickness, and it weighs from one ounce to an ounce and a half. The *fundus* is the upper broad extremity of the organ; it is convex, covered by peritoneum, and placed in a line below the level of the brim of the pelvis. The *body* gradually narrows from the fundus to the neck. Its anterior surface is flattened, covered by peritoneum in the upper three-fourths of its extent, and separated from the bladder by some convolutions of the small intestines; the lower fourth is connected with the bladder. Its posterior surface is convex, covered by peritoneum throughout, and separated from the rectum by some convolutions of the intestines. The lateral margins are concave, and give attachment to the Fallopian tubes above or superiorly, and the round ligaments below; and behind these, and also below the ligament of the ovary. The *cervix* is the lower and constricted portion of the uterus; around its circumference is attached the upper end of the vagina, and this extends upwards a greater distance behind than in front. At the vaginal extremity of the uterus is a transverse aperture, the OS UTERI, bounded by two lips, an anterior one which is thick, and a posterior one, narrow and long. The os uteri, or os tincæ, is generally about the size of a small goose-quill. The *canal of the cervix* is from half to three-quarters of an inch long; leading from the os uteri it first widens and then contracts again where it enters the body of the uterus. The surface of the canal exhibits a variable number of follicles or vesicles called the *glandula nabothi*, which secrete a thick mucus; this blocks the canal after impregnation. The cavity of the body and neck has a longitudinal extent of about two and a half inches; in virgins it is much less. (Fig. <u>12</u>).

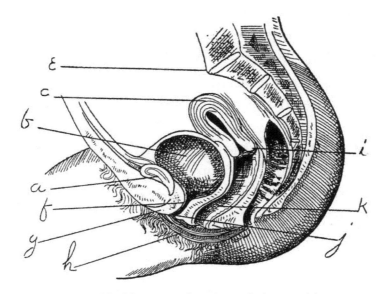

Fig. 11 Uterus, bladder, etc., showing relative position.

Fig. 11—Section of pelvis. a, section of pubis; b, bladder distended; c, the uterus in normal position; e, sacrum; f, urethra; g, vagina; h, hymen; i, the os uteri; j, meatus of urethra; k, vagina.

STRUCTURE OF THE UTERUS.

The proper tissue of the womb is composed of fibres, and is proved to be muscular. In the unimpregnated state it is dense, firm, and of a grayish color. The neck appears less firm than the body.

The *internal or mucous membrane* is thin, smooth, and closely adherent to the subjacent tissue. It is a quarter of an inch thick at the middle of the body of the uterus; in the neck it does not exceed one-twenty-fourth part of an inch in thickness. It is continuous through the fimbriated extremity of the Fallopian tubes with the peritoneum, and through the os uteri with the mucous membrane of the vagina.

THE FALLOPIAN TUBES.

The uterine or Fallopian tubes are two canals, about four inches long, placed in the superior border of the broad ligaments of the uterus. They extend for about three inches and a half, when they expand and terminate with a fringed process called the fimbria, which is applied to the ovary after impregnation. The Fallopian tubes serve the double purpose of a canal for transmitting the fecundating principle of the male and for carrying the germ furnished by the female to the uterus—in fact they are excretory ducts of the ovary.

Injections into the uterus may pass into the peritoneal cavity, through the Fallopian tubes, and cause peritonitis.

At each menstrual period an ovula passes along with the serum current in the Fallopian tubes to the uterus.

THE OVARIES.

The ovaries in the female are said to be the analogues of the testicles in the male; they both secrete a fluid that is essential to impregnation. They are situated on either side of the uterus, and are attached to either side of it by the posterior duplicature of the broad ligament called the ligament of the ovary. (Fig. 12).

They are oval flattened bodies about an inch and a half long, three-quarters of an inch wide at their greatest breadth, and a quarter of a inch thick. They are situated on the sides of the uterus in that portion of the broad ligament called the posterior wing, just behind the Fallopian tubes. The ovary consists of a peculiar structure enclosed by two envelopes, one of which is serous and the other fibrous. Within the fibrous coat is a special tissue called the stroma; imbedded in this are numerous small round transparent vesicles in various stages of development, varying in size from that of a millet seed to that of a hemp seed. They are the ovisacs, containing the ova, and are called the Graafian vesicles. These have thin transparent walls and contain a clear fluid, and within that the ovula. Fifteen or twenty may readily be distinguished in the adult female without the aid of magnifying glasses.

THE VAGINA.

The vagina is a membranous canal, extending from the vulva to the uterus obliquely through the pelvic cavity, between the bladder and rectum, having about the same direction as the axis of the pelvis. It is described as being five or six inches in length and about two inches in diameter, but it would be more correct to say that it is capable of being distended to these or greater dimensions, for in its common state the os uteri is seldom found to be more than three inches from the external orifice, and the vagina is contracted as well as shortened. In great part the walls of the vagina are composed of spongy erectile tissue, and their vascularity is a cause of considerable hemorrhage consequent on their rupture. Three layers combine to form the walls; one external or cellulo-fibrous, a middle or muscular one, and the internal or mucous one. The latter is of a pale red hue, which becomes violet during menstruation and especially during pregnancy. The mucous coat is disposed in the form of rugæ or folds anteriorly and posteriorly, which are better developed in young virgins and aged females;

during advanced pregnancy, and for a short time after delivery, they are entirely effaced.

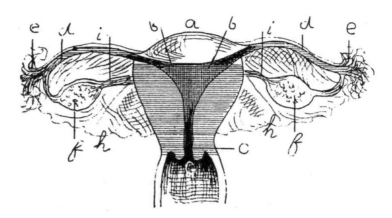

Fig. 12—Section of the Uterus, &c.

Fig. 12—Uterus, ovaries and Fallopian tubes. Section of the uterus, etc. a, Fundus of the uterus; b, cavity of the womb; c, cavity of the neck of the uterus; d, d, the cavity of the Fallopian tubes; e, fimbriated extremity; f, f, the ovaries; g, the vagina; h, h, the round ligaments; i, i, the ligaments of the ovaries.

The upper part of the vagina is connected to the circumference of the os uteri but not in a straight line, for the former stretches beyond the latter, and being joined to the cervix, its mucous membrane is reflected over the os uteri, which by this mode of union is suspended with protuberant lips in the vagina, and permitted to change its position in various ways and directions.

THE EXTERNAL ORGANS.

The situation of the external organs of generation are indicated in the accompanying diagram (Fig. 11.) It is not deemed necessary here to describe these, but in regard to the hymen (the membrane that in infancy nearly closes the orifice of the vagina), we may remark that it is not a perfect test of virginity. There are, however, examples recorded in works on midwifery where a slight surgical operation was necessary after marriage, because this membrane was uncommonly strong.

CHAPTER III.
PHYSIOLOGY OF THE UTERUS AND OVARIES.

Menstruation is a periodical flow of blood having its source in the walls of the uterus. But menstruation is excited by and dependent upon ovulation, and the effective cooperation of both the uterus and ovaries is necessary to both menstruation and conception. We shall consider these functions separately.

MENSTRUATION.

In healthy women at the period of puberty, a certain amount of sanguineous fluid is secreted by the lining membrane of the uterus, and is excreted through the vagina every month; this is termed the catamenia, or menses, and the function itself menstruation. A female in whom the discharge recurs at the usual periods, in the usual quantity, and of the usual quality, is said to be regular, The occurrence of menstruation defines the period of puberty at which a girl becomes a woman capable of conception, and its cessation terminates the prolific period of female life.

Dr. Robinson, of Manchester, England, in a paper on the natural history of menstruation, has stated the age at which it occurred in 450 cases.

According to his table, 10 menstruated for the first time at 11 years of age, 19 at 12, 53 at 13, 85 at 14, 97 at 15, 76 at 16, 57 at 17, 26 at 18, 23 at 19, and 4 at 20.

The time at which the first menstruation occurs varies exceedingly from the influence of climate, habits of life and constitution. There have been occasional instances of very precocious menstruation, in which the first appearance of the discharge was attended with all the attributes of puberty. I myself knew one case where a girl of nine years, not only menstruated, but presented the external signs of puberty, such as prominent breasts, wide pelvis, rounded contour of body, &c.

The first appearance of the menses very rarely occurs without being preceded by premonitory symptoms. There is usually a degree of languor and lassitude, fatigue after exertion, inequality of spirits, dark shade under the eyes, headache, sometimes pain in the thyroid gland, pain in the back, a sensation of tension and swelling in the lower part of the abdomen, and occasionally considerably fever. Not unfrequently strange nervous disturbances occur; but all of these symptoms may pass off, the first and second time, without the appearance of the menses, or with a white discharge only. Usually the phenomena may last from one to eight days, then there is an abundant flow of mucus, which after one or two days is mixed with blood, and soon gives place to almost pure blood. When this discharge takes place most of the unpleasant symptoms disappear, and the female only complains of weakness and is somewhat pale. The hemorrhage continues for several days, then the amount of blood mingled with the vaginal mucosities diminishes, soon there is mucus alone, then the discharge ceases.

I should remark now that the propriety of applying the terms, blood or hemorrhage, to the menstrual secretion is properly questioned.

Sometimes the first menstruation takes place without being preceded by any discomfort, but pretty generally there is a change in the girl at the time, both in her body and mind, a change that fits her for the important duties that devolve upon her.

Most young girls have a return of the discharge after a month, the menses afterwards recurring regularly; some do not become regular until after several months. Sometimes the function is imperfectly performed; such cases are accompanied with considerable distress.

In some young girls the precursory symptoms of the first appearance of the menses may not be followed by a flow of blood, and there is an apparent effort of nature recurring monthly for several months before the courses become established.

There are occasional examples of retarded menstruation. I am acquainted with one woman who at the age of twenty-five years has not menstruated. The absence of the menses does not render conception impossible, in every case.

After the menses are established, until the time of their cessation, they generally return every month, unless interrupted by pregnancy or nursing.

The average of the catamenial period is about twenty-eight days; in a large number it is thirty days; in some instances they recur every fifteen days.

The duration of the flow varies from one to eight days; three or four days is the most usual duration. The quantity of blood lost is variable; from three to five ounces is said to be the average.

When the ovaries are congenitally absent, or have been removed, or have become disorganized, menstruation is absent, or ceases. The cause of the menses is the successive evolution of the Graafian vesicles; but the regular process may go on in the ovary without the regular sanguineous discharge.

The menses continue in the majority of cases until about the age of 46 years, or perhaps in this country 48 years.

According to Dr. Robertson, of England, the periods at which it closed in 77 individuals was, in 1 at the age of 35 years, 4 at 40, 1 at 42, 1 at 43, 3 at 44, 4 at 45, 3 at 47, 10 at 48, 7 at 49, 26 at 50, 2 at 51, 2 at 52, 2 at 53, 2 at 54, 1 at 57, 2 at 60, and 1 at 70.

The average duration of the menstrual function is about 30 years. The cessation of the ovarian function is generally announced several years in advance by irregularities of the menses. Besides the intermissions and irregularities, there are other symptoms; a general and indefinite feeling of uneasiness, pelvic pains, itching at the genital parts, flashes of heat in the face, alterations of chilliness and perspiration, leucorrhœa, etc. These troubles are usually slight, and disappear promptly. The time of life has been called the CRITICAL PERIOD, because there has been an opinion prevalent that peculiar dangers attend it. However, the mortality is not greater between the ages of 45 and 50 years than at any other period of life. Yet it is true that in some instances diseases that had been latent previously, declare themselves at this period.

THE FUNCTION OF THE OVARIES.

We will now consider the physiological action of the ovaries and its intimate connection with the action of the uterus in menstruation, etc.

Preceding the first menstruation an ovary is considerably enlarged, becomes of a red color, and its vascular apparatus is considerably congested; the Fallopian tube also becomes congested; its fimbriated extremity is of a violet red color, and has a velvety appearance. The Graafian vesicles increase in size; fifteen or twenty of them, more advanced than the others, project from the surface of the ovary; one of these grows so that after a few days it forms a tumor of the size of a cherry; the walls of the vesicle, being distended by an increased secretion of fluid, becomes quite thin, and at last are ruptured. When the thinned walls give way, the ovule is expelled, with a part of the granular contents of the vesicle; these are grasped by the fimbriated extremity of the Fallopian tube which is prepared to receive it and convey it through its canal into the cavity of the uterus.

This evolution of an ovule excites numerous sympathies throughout the organism of the female, and especially the generative organs. The vascular apparatus of the womb becomes developed in an unusual manner; a network of fine blood vessels surround the orifices of the numerous glandular tubes, of which the membrane is almost entirely composed; this gives a violet hue to the internal surface of the womb; the utricular glands increase in size, the muscular structure of the uterus acquires greater extension, becomes redder and more spongy and supple, the volume of the organ is increased, the neck is tumefied and its orifice narrower, the lips of the os tincæ are warmer and their color deeper.

The vascular congestion which the uterus undergoes is accompanied with the exudation of sanguineous fluid, which is at first but a few drops; this communicates to the increased vaginal mucus a reddish hue. After a day or two there is a bloody flow from the vascular network of the mucous membrane. This flow, which constitutes the menses, is diminished after three or four days, and the discharge again contains a large proportion of mucus and serum. It is probable that the rupture of a Graafian vesicle occurs during the last days of the flow, ordinarily, and it is also believed that venereal excitement is capable of exerting so much influence upon it that it may determine the rupture of an enlarged vesicle, which, without sexual intercourse, would have remained whole several days longer.

After the discharge of the ovule consequent on the rupture of the Graafian vesicle, the walls of the vesicle contract on the matter that is effused within it, and form a compact mass, which after a time has an orange yellow color—this is called the *corpus luteum*.

Ordinarily, in the human female in the normal condition, a new Graafian vesicle increases in size every month, becomes excessively developed, and finally bursts and discharges its ovule, to become, through successive transformations, the *corpus luteum*. What is called the "monthly sickness," "monthlies," "courses," etc., never occurs without having been preceded and accompanied by the development of a Graafian vesicle.

CHAPTER IV.
OF DISPLACEMENTS OF THE UTERUS.

In order to compress as much as possible what I say upon these topics, I shall consider here displacements of the uterus, both of those which occur in the pregnant and non-pregnant women.

By the inflection of the peritoneum the uterus is permitted to expand freely during pregnancy, and to rise without inconvenience into the cavity of the abdomen; this it could not do if it was confined to its place by short ligaments, or by adhesions. But from the same cause, women become liable to various diseases; to the retroversion of the uterus, and other displacements; to dropsy of the peritoneum, and to that species of hernia which is occasioned by the descent of the intestines between the vagina and rectum.

By PROLAPSIS is meant that condition in which the uterus falls below its natural level in the pelvic cavity. PROCIDENTIA is a term used to signify the protrusion of the uterus beyond the vulva. Women are liable, even when young, to a falling of the womb, but it occurs most commonly after the age of thirty-five, in such as lead a laborious life. Amongst other causes may be enumerated violent bearing down efforts, such as are made in straining to pass hardened feces, or in urging an evacuation through a stricture in the rectum, in coughing, lifting heavy weights, etc.

The immediate causes of the displacements are the pressure on the uterus by the viscera above it, and a diminution in tone of the uterine supports.

Displacements of the womb are more common among women who have hollow and capacious pelves; in sufferers from dropsy, and in delicate, flabby subjects, where the broad and round ligaments are affected and elongated.

There may be prolapsis during the early months of pregnancy, and in cases where the pelvis is large and the ligaments are relaxed, the womb may rest on the perineum; or the neck, and even the body may become visible externally; but it subsequently rises out of the pelvic cavity, assuming a normal position.

When a woman has prolapsis uteri she often complains of a sense of weight about the pelvis, of dragging pains, of a wearisome backache, and of a leucorrhocal discharge. Menstruation is seldom interfered with, and as the uterus goes back of itself, or is easily pushed up when the patient is in bed, conception may take place, and the general health may not be directly affected.

In some few instances there is complete inability to pass water until the patient lies down and replaces the uterus with her finger; in other cases micturition may be annoyingly frequent. Constipation is often complained of, and, if the woman be careless, a large accumulation of feces may take place in the rectum.

By a vaginal examination the os uteri is found low down, and if the cervix is of the natural length, we know that it is prolapsis.

If a round tumor is seen projecting beyond the vulva, and if at the lowest part of it there is what seems to be the mouth of the uterine cavity, it may be advisable to introduce a sound or catheter, to make sure that the opening is not a mere cleft in a uterine polypus. (Of course, you would not use a sound if you suspected pregnancy.) If there are ulcers, cracks, etc., they may be detected, the ulcers looking as if portions of the mucous lining had been punched out.

In pregnancy, displacements may occur either slowly or suddenly, though the woman may have had nothing of the kind previously, or they may be the continuation of a previous prolapse. The progressive development of the uterus generally removes the prolapsis about the fourth or fifth month, but if the pelvis is very large, it may possibly continue.

As in other cases of prolapsis, the pregnant woman may suffer very much from it. She may suffer from a feeling of weight at the anus; painful tractions in the groins, lumber regions and umbilicus; a fetid discharge may come on; there may be complete retention of urine, very obstinate constipation, etc.; and the pressure on the uterus may cause abortion.

For complete retention of the urine the catheter may be used, or the womb may be pressed up by one or two fingers introduced into the vagina; or the woman may be able to urinate if she lies down and elevates her hips considerably.

THE OPERATION OF INTRODUCING THE CATHETER may be performed by the educated nurse. The patient being placed upon her back and the labia separated, the point of the forefinger of the left hand should be placed just within the orifice of the vagina so as to press slightly the upper edge; the catheter should then be passed along the inner surface of the finger until it is arrested by the anterior part of the vagina; when there, a very slight movement so as to elevate the point of the instrument a little, enables the operator in the majority of cases to enter the catheter into the canal. The operation is more difficult when the parts are swollen or distended, as happens occasionally from disease, during pregnancy or labor, or after delivery. If we cannot detect the orifice by the touch, we may use a light, and the patient may be placed on her side. We may adopt another way to proceed. The point of the forefinger finds the clitoris, and passes from above downwards to the middle of the vestibule; the first inequality met with is the orifice of the urethra, into which the instrument can then be passed. It will easily slide in if the instrument is not passed either to the right or the left of the median line.

When a woman who has previously suffered from prolapsis becomes pregnant, it is sometimes necessary for her to keep the horizontal position during the first three or four months of pregnancy, and after her confinement she should keep her bed a considerable time—perhaps for two months.

For the treatment of prolapsis in non-pregnant women, the general principles are to be applied: To afford artificial support to the superincumbent abdominal viscera; give tone to the broad and round ligaments of the uterus, to the vaginal walls and the perineum; and to remove any complications that induce the falling, such as uterine congestion, hypertrophy, cough, constipation, etc.

The uterus may usually be easily pushed back to its place when the patient is lying down, or, what is better, her head much lower than her pelvis. (Fig. 13). The knee-chest position is the best one.

Without going into the details of treatment in the use of bandages, tents, etc., I may say that a nurse may, in the absence of a physician, use astringent vaginal injections, astringent pessaries (F. 154, 163), and cold soft water; hip baths may also be used. The nurse should know how to tamponade the vagina, because, when this is deemed advisable by the physician, he desires that the process be repeated every day, and in many instances it is not convenient or possible for him to make daily visits. The vaginal tampon is used as a means of retaining the uterus in its normal position, and also to hold medicinal agents applied to the cervix and vagina; besides, in some cases, direct pressure on the pelvic vessels stimulates and thus benefits them when in a state of chronic, passive dilatation, or venous hyperemia. Tampons are also used in cases of hemorrhage from the uterus, and as an absorbent of vaginal or uterine discharges, and for various other purposes.

The nurse may receive instruction from the physician in each case in regard to the material, etc., to be used as tampon. When it is desired to simply support the uterus in its place, fine cotton batting may be used, and this perhaps is, in ordinary cases, as good as any material. But in some cases absorbent cotton, oakum, marine lint, or wool may be preferred. The size of the tampon will, of course, vary; ordinarily one as large as a hen's egg may be introduced without difficulty; sometimes one nearly as large as a goose egg may be necessary, because a small one would not be retained. Cotton may be rolled tightly into the form of a cylinder, or a small bag may be made of muslin or linen, and cotton or other substance can be enclosed in this and applied.

The knee-pectoral position (Fig. 13) is the one in which a prolapsed uterus can best be replaced, and the nurse can best tamponade the vagina while the patient is in that position. The *proper* knee-pectoral or knee-chest position is shown in Fig. 13.

The physician would, with or without the aid of the nurse, use a Sims' speculum, and first pack four small pledgets of cotton around the neck of the uterus. One string can be tied in the kite-tail manner around each of these pledgets, and there should be an end about ten inches long to be left out from the vagina, so that the whole may be easily removed. The nurse, if alone, however, will usually press in but one tampon, and she may do this while the patient is in the knee-chest position, or, what is nearly as well, on her side or back, having first, by a digital examination, ascertained that the uterus is in its proper position.

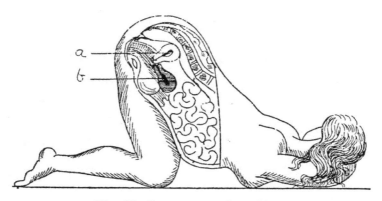

Fig. 13. Genu-pectoral position.

Fig. 13—Knee-chest or genu-pectoral position.

a,   Retroversion of the uterus.

b,   Natural position of the uterus.

Either the nurse or the patient herself may easily press a tampon into its proper position, if she possesses an ordinary amount of boldness and dexterity. She will find it more difficult to properly place it, however, if there is tannin or other astringent substance on the outside of it. This has an astringent effect immediately when it comes in contact with the vagina, and an unusual amount of vaseline is necessary to cover it.

If a solution of tannin, alum, acetate of lead, sulphate of zinc, or carbolic acid be used, it is best to prepare several tampons at the same time; soak all the tampons in the solution, squeeze them out and dry them, then when one is used put it inside a bag and apply it dry.

The patient herself, if she is intelligent, and is not too timid, can introduce the tampon. She should first smear its surface with vaseline, lard, or olive oil. Then lying on her back with thighs separated and flexed, draw the labia apart with the fingers of one hand and steadily crowd the tampon into the vagina with the other, always taking care to have a good, strong cord, one end attached to the tampon and the other hanging down to facilitate removal.

It is well also, sometimes, to place another pledget of cotton between the labia, that can be removed when the woman urinates. When all is well crowded into place, the tampon should be retained by a broad T bandage, covered by oiled silk when it rests against the vulva.

Generally the whole should be removed within from eighteen to twenty-four hours, and hot water or some cleansing injection used, and the tampon be soon reapplied.

If opium or morphine is used with the tampon, as it is sometimes when there is considerable pain, first dip the cotton in glycerine, and then sprinkle the narcotic on the outside.

If borax, tannin, alum, acetate of lead, sulphate of zinc, chlorate of potash, or carbolic acid is used, I think it well to envelop the undissolved drug in cotton, put it in the middle of the tampon, and let it dissolve slowly in the vagina. It is best when thus applied to let the whole suppository remain as much as forty-eight hours; it should, however, be removed when it seems to cause smarting or excoriations.

The accompanying cut (Fig. 13) is inserted to show what is the knee-chest or genu-pectoral position, as well as to exhibit the retroversion of the uterus. Note that in this position the hips are elevated, and remember that it does not suffice to get on the hands and knees if the haunches are low down on the legs and ankles.

RETROFLEXION AND ANTIFLEXION.

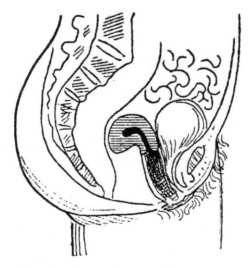

Fig. 14. Retroflexion of the uterus.

The condition known as *retroflexion* consists of a bending back of the uterus at a point where the neck joins the body, so that the fundus is found between the cervix and rectum, the os uteri being in the natural position.

In *antiflexion* we find the fundus pressing upon the bladder. These displacements are rare in virgins. The false membrane formed in peritonitis is now and then the cause of these deviations, when there is superadded such causes as are mentioned for prolapsis. The symptoms of RETROFLEXION are usually a dull, weary and constant backache, which is more marked about the sacral region, pains that shoot down the thighs or the groins, and a frequent desire to go to stool, although nothing comes away. The passage of a motion that is not at all constipated aggravates the pain and aching; sexual intercourse is attended with suffering, and is not followed by pregnancy; and just before and after the monthly periods there is so much tenderness that sexual connection cannot be tolerated.

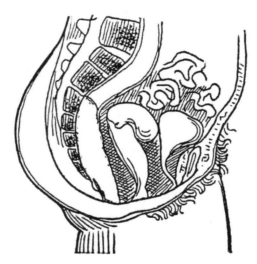

Fig. 15. Antiflexion of the uterus.

The catamenia come on with pain and difficulty, but about the second day the flow of blood seems to give some relief. The general health is bad, there are frequent attacks of nausea, the appetite is small, the spirits are depressed, and there are many what are called hysterical symptoms. On examination the congested fundus may be found encroaching upon the rectum; on touching this part the patient will exclaim that it is the seat of her sufferings, and it is not uncommon to find tenderness of one or both ovaries.

Not many of these symptoms are present in ANTIFLEXION, but this commonly produces great irritability of the bladder, so that when the patient is in the erect position, the desire to micturate is almost as great as in disease of the bladder.

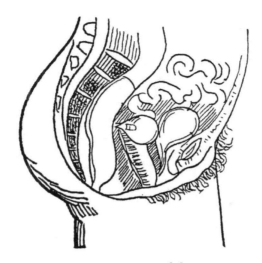

Fig. 16. Anteversion of the uterus.

The treatment includes replacing the uterus with the sound. Should there be adhesions, however, this might cause intolerable pain. In such cases relief is given by the use of belladonna plasters and belladonna, opium, hyoscyamus, or conium tampons. One-half to one dram of the tincture of one of the narcotics may be added to the glycerine in which the tampon is soaked, or the cervical end of the tampon may be dipped in the tincture. Suppositories and ointments may also be used. (F. 163, 214).

RETROVERSION AND ANTEVERSION.

In RETROVERSION (Fig. 13) the fundus is turned toward the hollow of the sacrum, while the os is drawn under the arch of the pubis.

ANTEVERSION is characterized by the fundus being towards or against the bladder, the os being directed to the cavity of the sacrum. (Fig. 16.) Retroversion is liable to occur at the third month of pregnancy, from the neglected distention of the bladder, and from a morbid weight and enlargement, though after the fourth month the uterus is too much enlarged to fall down in any way. The chief symptoms are backache and bearing down pains. It may happen that micturation will be impeded; and if the bladder may be felt at the lower part of the abdomen, or if the patient complain of a constant desire to pass water, or especially if the urine should dribble away, the catheter ought to be passed without loss of time, and the bladder should be kept evacuated. It may be necessary, in order to restore the organ to its proper position, to introduce the first and second fingers of one hand into the vagina, and a finger of the other into the rectum.

CHAPTER V.
MISMENSTRUATION.

AMENORRHŒA.

The first variety of cases of amenorrhœa are those where no menstrual fluid has ever been secreted. All girls, as we have seen, do not menstruate at fifteen years, as all children do not cut their first teeth at seven months, and in either case there may be no disease. But when a female has reached adult life, when her frame has assumed the character of womanhood, when she is not chlorotic, and when all her organs (save the sexual) perform their functions naturally, then a cause of the absence of the flux should be looked for. Menstruation may be absent from congenital malformation. The ovaries may be wanting, or if present may be atrophied or diseased; perhaps they present scarcely a trace of a Graafian vesicle; or these glands can exist and the uterus be absent or imperfect; or there may not be found a trace of a vagina. In the second variety of amenorrhœa there has been a secretion of the menses but no evacuation of them. This may be because there is an occlusion of the vagina, or the os uteri may be imperforate. When the os is closed by a membrane, the structure may be incised with the bistoury, or perhaps be ruptured by the uterine sound.

The third variety is the most common form of amenorrhœa, viz: that in which the flux having been properly established and appearing regularly for a time, has been prematurely arrested. But it may be said of amenorrhœa in its various forms, that it is not so much a disease as a symptom of disease; a consequence of either individual organization, disorder of the uterus or ovaries, or of some other organ or organs sufficiently important to affect the constitution.

Hence all the means that restore the system to health, medicinal and hygienic, may be recommended as tending to cure the complaint, and hence we have to inquire whether there is serious disease in any of the organs when the question of pregnancy arises, on account of the disappearance of the menses.

It is always necessary in treating amenorrhœa to consider the cause of it, and we should know that it may come from torpitude of the secernent vessels of the uterus, produced by anxiety of mind, cold, or suddenly suppressed perspiration; falls, especially when accompanied with terror; or a general inertness and flaccidity of the system, and more particularly of the ovaries. (F. 172, 173).

DYSMENORRHŒA.

There are few women who pass through the whole period of sexual vigor without having more or less frequently to endure an attack of dysmenorrhœa. Some few females experience great pain with each flow, from puberty to the change of life, while in others pain is only an exceptional accompaniment. With some women marriage effects a cure, while in others it either aggravates or originates dysmenorrhœa. Three distinct varieties of dysmenorrhœa have to be considered: the neuralgic, the congestive, and the mechanical.

The variety which is called NEURALGIC DYSMENORRHŒA is more frequent in unmarried females; and if married, in those that have not borne children; and most frequently affects those of a nervous temperament, and of a thin, delicate habit. The paroxysms present all the characteristics of neuralgia. For a time before the catamenia appear there is a sense of general uneasiness, a deep-seated feeling of cold and headache, sometimes alternating with pain in the back and lower part of the abdomen, perhaps extending down the thighs.

The flux comes on sometimes slowly and scantily, or in some cases in slight gushes. The discharge may be paler than natural, and may be mixed with slight clots. In some cases there is a membrane of plastic lymph discharged either in shreds, or in the form of the uterine cavity that it has lined. Conception is rare under such circumstances.

Though the disease seems to be of a simple neuralgic character, it is supposed that there is a degree of inflammation of a peculiar kind in the mucous membrane where the plastic lymph is thrown off.

In regard to the duration of the period, the constitutional injury sustained, and as to the relief on the appearance of the menses, the cases vary.

A peculiar irritability of the uterus is a common cause of this form of the disease, but, like amenorrhœa, it may be caused by cold, mental emotion, or local injury from a fall.

In the treatment of this class of cases, to reduce the pain, opium, conium, hyoscyamus, etc., are given, often combined with camphor. (F. 161, 163, 166, 167.) These should be given in the form of an enema, or a suppository, if the stomach is irritable. (F. 160.) The hot hip bath should be employed, the patient remaining in it from thirty-five to forty minutes; an ounce of carbonate of soda may be added to the water. The good effects of the bath may be kept up by the use, immediately afterwards, of a pessary of oxide of zinc and belladonna. (F. 163.) It will be of benefit to take vaginal injections of tepid, or warm, or hot water on the approach of the menses, and the patient should use a pediluvium, or a hip bath, for two or three nights in succession antecedent to the show of the menses. During the interval every effort should be made to strengthen the patient, and to diminish the irritability. Injections of tepid or cold water may be taken daily; the diet should be nourishing, and plenty of exercise in the open air should be taken by the patient. Some preparation of iron should be given, and I have found F. 177 particularly useful.

CONGESTIVE DYSMENORRHŒA, sometimes described as *inflammatory* dysmenorrhœa, generally comes on at a later time of life than the neuralgic form. It occurs in females of a full habit and of a sanguine temperament; in the married as well as the unmarried, and those that have not borne children.

Restlessness and feverishness, rigors, flushing and headache generally precede the severer symptoms. The sufferings commence, or are generally aggravated four or five days before the period, and it may continue for a week or more. Both before and after the catamenia appear, there is great pain across the back, aching of the limbs, intolerance of light and sound, weariness, the face is flushed, the skin hot, the pulse full and bounding; when the flow gets abundant the pain is mitigated, though there are paroxysms of pain, as small clots and shreds of membrane are thrown off from the uterine cavity. Under the influence of inflammation, the epithelial coat of the uterine cavity and of the vagina is sometimes expelled. In the interim between the periods the cervix uteri is congested and tender, and pain will be excited by pressing the ovaries; usually there is a tenacious leucorrhœal discharge. Frequently the breasts swell and become tender as the period approaches.

In treating this form of dysmenorrhœa, opiates must be used, as in the former variety, to afford some alleviation. Give also saline purgatives, febrifuge medicines, such as aconite, veratrium, and gelsemium; also cooling drinks. During the interval the patient should live plainly, avoid stimulants, and take moderate outdoor exercise. The suppositories (F. 163) may be used steadily. If the disease be associated with a rheumatic diathesis, the appropriate remedy for that should be used. It is in such cases especially that chalybeate mineral water, warm sea water, baths, colchicum, iodide of potassium, with friction and electricity applied directly to the hypogastric region, succeed in restoring health. (F. 103, 165).

MECHANICAL DYSMENORRHŒA is that form in which there is some mechanical obstruction to the escape of the menstrual discharge. The causes of the obstruction are various. There may be either a stricture of the internal orifice of the uterus, or a narrowing of the whole canal of the cervix, or the external os uteri may be small and contracted, or some tumor may interfere with the patency of the cervical canal, and there may be retroflexion or antiflexion of the uterus.

In these cases there is more or less violent expulsive pain coming on in paroxysms, and there is usually a scanty flow. Often the discharge escapes in gushes, each gush being preceded by a bearing down effort, and accompanied by an expulsive pain. There are attacks of nausea, restlessness and retching, with flatulence; there is always severe headache and congestion, with tenderness of the ovaries; and if there is endometritis, there are some other inflammatory symptoms.

Modern gynecology has various remedies for this class of cases, of which it is not necessary to speak here.

MENORRHAGIA.

The term menorrhagia should be applied only to cases of menstrual flow, although it is often employed to signify any considerable sanguineous discharge from the uterus, other than normal monthly escape. But I will say something here of cases where there is a more abundant or a more prolonged flow than is natural to the subject of it, and of cases where there is a recurrence of the discharge at short intervals, so as to seem almost continuous.

In that variety in which the discharge is normal in quality but the quantity is increased, there is undue uterine congestion, set up by constitutional causes, or it is induced by slight disease of the uterus or ovaries.

When menorrhagia takes place in plethoric habits, it is manifestly remedial, and ought not to be restrained hastily. We may endeavor to reduce the plethora, and a cooling diet, the recumbent position, and saline cathartics may be enjoined. (F. 61).

If the flow continues five days or more, and especially if depressing effects are manifested, such as general weakness, languor, mental depression, with pain in the head, loins or back, the patient is undoubtedly suffering from the loss of blood, and it is best to restrain the flux by general and local means (F. 176.) At the time when the flow is profuse or long continued, give strong cinnamon tea, a teacupful at a time, or teaspoonful doses of tincture cinnamon every hour. Astringent pessaries should sometimes be used. Formerly injections of cold water were given; recently injections of hot water, as hot as can be borne in the vagina, are considered more effectual. Fluid extract of ergot, in half-teaspoonful doses, may be given every hour for two or three successive hours. Other remedies are elixir vitriol and turpentine, opium and acetate of lead during the attack; and counter irritation to the sacrum, the douche to the loins, sponging, cold vaginal injections, and the sitz bath during the interval. (F. 175).

If astringent or cold injections are used, the patient should lie upon her back in bed, and the fluid should be thrown up gradually. Of course, there are cases where only an experienced, well-educated physician can do all that is required in removing the cause of the difficulty.

CHAPTER VI.
GENERATION.

Generation is effected in the human species through the medium of the two sexes; to effect it there must be the actual contact of the male semen, or its spermatozoa, with a healthy Graafian vesicle.

In CONCEPTION the SPERMATIC FLUID is furnished by the male. When this is examined under the microscope it exhibits a great number of little bodies, which are moving; these are termed spermatic animalcules, or spermatozoa. These are met with in all animals capable of reproduction, and they do not appear in the human species before puberty.

The ovule furnished by the female is existent in the ovary at the marriageable period. Fecundation takes place in the ovary; probably, sometimes, also in the tube or uterus when the ovule is passing out after menstruation.

Ordinarily the fluid ejaculated by the male must reach the uterus, and in some way be conveyed to the ovaries through the Fallopian tubes to produce fecundation.

It is believed that, as the consequence of copulation, the semen is thrown on the neck of the uterus; that it is carried forward, first, by the movements proper to the uterus and tubes; second, by the movements proper to the spermatozoa till it reaches the ovum, generally in the ovary; that it enters the ovum, and that then fecundation takes place.

Upon being impregnated and the vesicle bursting, the ovum is grasped by the free extremity of the Fallopian tubes, which is in contact with the ovary, the ovum passes from the ovary to the canal, is pressed onwards by the peristaltic motions of the tube through the duct, and finally reaches the uterine cavity; there it continues to grow during the ordinary term of gestation. After two hundred and seventy days the ovule has developed into a child, and is expelled through the natural parts of generation. When gestation proceeds in this manner, it is said to be normal, or good, or uterine; sometimes (though very seldom) the ovule is arrested at some point in its passage, and is developed outside of the womb; this is termed an *extra uterine pregnancy*.

The time at which conception is most likely to occur is that immediately following the flow of the menses; it may take place immediately before the flow, and sexual intercourse may be fruitful even when it takes place in the middle of the interval between the sexual periods, though the latter is unusual.

When conception takes place a few days or a few hours before the period, it is not followed by the menstrual flow.

UTERO-GESTATION.

At each menstrual period the bulk or size of the uterus is for the time increased, and if conception takes place about that time, the excitement maintains and soon increases the enlargement. The mucous membrane becomes almost doubled in thickness, and when the ovule arrives in the womb, it finds it filled with the membrane, the whole uterus is congested, its vessels enlarge, and are filled with blood, many which were invisible before are now filled with red blood, and the whole form an intricate network on the surface, and in the substance of the organ; the coats of the arteries increase in thickness; the coats of veins are thinner, and admit of still greater distention; the nerves increase in size, and may be seen accompanying the blood-vessels, and there are changes not only in the volume, but in the shape, situation, direction, and relations of the uterus.

The organ increases slowly in size during the early. months of pregnancy, and more rapidly in the later. The walls are distended, however, not mechanically from the development of the ovum, but simultaneously with it, and from a physiological cause; in shape it becomes rounder, and towards the end of pregnancy it has an ovoid form. Simultaneously there is an alteration in its position; at first the neck subsides towards the floor of the pelvis; the presence of the rectum may incline the fundus to the right and the neck to the left; about the fourth month the uterus rises above the superior strait; at four months the fundus uteri is two or three fingers in breadth above the pubis; at five months it is within one finger's breadth of the umbilicus; between the fifth and sixth month it passes the umbilicus; at seven months it is three fingers' breadth above the naval; at eight months it is four or five above, but it does not rise higher during the last month. While it is rising it follows the direction of the axis of the superior strait; afterwards it inclines to the right oftener than to the left.

At term, the superior part of the uterus is in contact with the abdominal walls usually, but sometimes there may be some of the intestines interposed between them.

At full term the parietes of the womb are thicker than in the unimpregnated condition; at the point corresponding to the insertion of the placenta, thinner at the neck, and otherwise it retains about its original thickness.

The uterus increases about forty times in weight during pregnancy; at term it weighs about twenty-four ounces, and its length is from twelve to fourteen inches, its breadth from nine to ten, and its depth, antero-posteriorly, eight to nine inches.

The os uteri, after it is in the gravid state, becomes somewhat swollen, but soft and cushion-like. This softening is at first superficial. Towards the end of the third month, the lips of the os tincæ are softened throughout their whole thickness, and the softening increases from below upward.

The *neck of the uterus* seems somewhat elongated at the first, but at the commencement of the sixth month the length of the cervix seems to diminish; there is, however, no considerable shortening until the middle of the eighth month; during the last fortnight of pregnancy it diminishes very rapidly, and finally is totally effaced.

In primapara the os tincæ is rounded at first, and is not dilated. In females that have had children the external orifice is widely open, and the cavity in the neck is funnel-shaped, continuing to increase until it reaches the internal orifice.

As gestation progresses the texture of the uterus changes. The peritoneum spreads out in all directions without a decrease in thickness; the mucous coat becomes apparent, it grows redder and more vascular, and its folds disappear; the glands of the body of the womb grow longer; the middle coat is enlarged by the increase in size of always existing muscular elements, and the formation of new fibres and increased connective tissue. There is, towards the end of pregnancy, an astonishing development of the vascular system; the lymphatic vessels acquire considerable calibre, and the nerves are developed in every way, although the neurilemma is most affected.

The changes developed in the uterine mucous membrane are of especial interest. Its vascularity is greatly increased during menstruation, the glands are enlarged, the membrane thickened, thrown into folds and becomes of a violet color; this condition continuing until the ovule is discharged, or until the last of the menstrual period. The fecundation of the ovum will maintain and increase this vascular condition of the membrane. Its vessels are so enlarged as to cause small effusions beneath the epithelium, which gives to the internal surface a spotted appearance; after two or three weeks it is still more mottled, more puffed up, and furrowed with folds and wrinkles. This membrane is the *decidua*, which is afterwards expelled, with other contents of the uterine cavity.

The DECIDUA REFLEXA is a fold of the decidua in which the fœtus is enveloped, and both of these membranes, which are at the last expelled with the fœtus, are developed from the uterine mucous membrane. The uterine decidua, after the second month, grows thinner, and its folds are gradually effaced; after the fifth month it is only one twenty-fifth of an inch in thickness, and it is still thinner at the termination of pregnancy. At the fifth month it is separable from the uterus, and the first trace of the new membrane which is to replace the decidua may be detected under it. A partly uterine membrane may be thrown off when an abortion occurs, during the early months of pregnancy.

CHAPTER VII.
THE OVUM AND ITS DEVELOPMENT.

The ovum at maturity (and not impregnated) is described as being composed of the vitelline membrane, which seems like albumen in appearance, but is a thick, transparent membrane, without determinate texture; second of the vitellus or yolk, a granular liquid contained in the vitelline membrane, composed of a coherent transparent viscid mass; third of the germinal vesicle, which is composed of a transparent colorless membrane, enclosing a liquid also transparent; and lastly, of the germinal spot, that is held in suspension in the liquid that the germinal vesicle contains.

The ovum passes slowly through the Fallopian tubes, and during the twelve days or more that it is passing to the uterus, there is some development, some increase in size, and by the time it has reached the uterus it has become impossible to find in it either vesicle or germinal spot.

It is probable that in its passage it is nourished by the granulations which accompany it, and by absorbing the liquid secreted by the oviduct.

As the impregnated ovum is developed, the chorion, the amnion and the embryo may be observed.

The *chorion*, which corresponds to the membrane lining in the shell of an egg, is found covering the ovum at the earliest period that it has been seen in the uterus. It is smooth internally, but externally it is covered with short round villi, which at a later period remain only where the placenta is developed. The chorion is enveloped in a great measure by the reflected decidua; there is at the outset considerable space between the two, mostly filled at first by the villi of the chorion, though there may be between the two an effusion of blood; these villi soon disappear, and the membranes come in contact.

In that part of the chorion that is not covered by the decidua reflexa, the villi are more and more developed, and they contribute a most important part in the formation of the placenta.

At the same time that the placenta is formed, the villi on the other portion of the chorion is obliterated, so that the principal part of the chorion is a thin, colorless, transparent membrane, united outwardly to the reflexed decidua by short, delicate filaments, and inwardly to the amnion by an albuminous layer called the *tunica media*.

There is also between the two membranes the *vesicula alba*. This bears a perfect analogy to the yolk of an egg; it is the vitellus surrounded by the blastoderm. Its use is to contain nutriment for the fœtus before the development of the placenta.

The amnion is the most internal membrane of the ovum; it is continuous with the margins of the ventral opening in the fœtus, and closely envelopes the embryo in the early period. Its internal surface exhales a liquid into its own internal cavity, and in this the embryo swims freely.

As this membrane is more and more filled, it presses back the exterior liquid and thereby condenses it until the amnion comes in contact with the chorion. And since it adheres to the abdominal parietes of the fœtus, it furnishes as it extends a membranous sheath to the allantoid and umbilical vesicle, and these vessels, and all parts thus enclosed constitute the *umbilical* cord.

The *placenta* is an appendage of the chorion; it is a soft, spongy mass, constituting the principal connection between the ovum and the uterus, being destined to the hematosis and (as we suppose) to the nourishment of the fœtus. The placenta, at the termination of utero gestation, is a flattened body about an inch in thickness at the center; its shape is circular or oval, and it is from six to eight and one-half inches in diameter; its internal surface is covered by the chorion and amnion, and exhibits plainly the umbilical arteries and veins which converge to form the umbilical cord. Its fœtal portion is formed by the hypertrophied villi of the chorion, with which its circumference is continuous, and its maternal portion is continuous with the decidua, and is in fact a thickened part of that membrane. As the villi of the chorion are developed on one part of its surface, they ramify and form filaments that engraft themselves upon the uterine mucous membrane and adhere closely. At the same time there is an inverse development of the uterine vessels, which form vast numbers of loops that descend between the villi of the chorion, and extend through to the fœtal surface of the placenta. An amorphous matter is soon thrown out which unites the two parts together.

The placenta is, therefore, composed of two parts, distinct in their physiological action, though they together present but one mass to our view. One part is the fœtal portion formed from the chorion; the other is the maternal portion formed from the uterine mucous membrane, of which it is a greatly thickened part. After delivery the fœtal placenta comes entirely away with the epithelial layer of the placental decidua, and the placental distribution of the maternal vessels; a portion of the maternal vessels remains attached to the uterus.

The placenta may be inserted upon any part of the uterine cavity, although it is most usually near the fundus where the ovum must enter the womb. If, as is sometimes the case, it is attached at the lower part, over the orifice of the womb, it causes unavoidable hemorrhage in the later months of pregnancy.

The *umbilical cord, funis, or naval string,* is the connecting link between the child and mother. It commences when the external lamina of the blastoderm with the alantois are so changed as to form a mere cord upon which the two umbilical arteries ramify, and when all these have an enveloping sheath from the amnios. It may be discerned in this state at the end of the first month; at that time the fœtal intestines may be seen to protrude beyond the umbilicus into the amnionic sheath, but the cord is then cylindrical and very small. There are progressive changes, the cord becomes simplified, the canal of the amnionic sheath is obliterated gradually at its extremity, and as the effacement proceeds towards the umbilicus the intestine is pressed back so that no hernia remains.

There are two arteries in the cord; these arise from the abdominal aorta in the fœtus; they go by a flexed and tortuous course to the placenta, where they ramify and are distributed. There is only one vein which returns the blood from the placenta; there the radicles coalesce to form the branches; these unite to form the umbilical vein. This is not as flexuous as the arteries, which, being longer, wind around the one venous trunk. After the third month these may be plainly seen in the sheath imbedded in what has been called *Wharton's gellatine.*

Ordinarily the cord lies free and loose in the cavity of the amnion, but occasionally owing to the movements of the child it may be coiled around the child's neck, be tied in knots, or it may escape below the head so as to prolapse during labor.

The length of the cord varies; it is very rarely less than eight inches, and it is sometimes six or eight feet long.

After the birth of the child, the pulsation in the cord ceases within about fifteen minutes. After the cord is cut that portion that is attached to the umbilicus dies and usually falls off about the fifth day.

The blood of the fœtus is ærated or undergoes a change in the placenta analagous to the change that our blood undergoes in the lungs.

CHAPTER VIII.
THE FŒTUS.

The embryo first begins to be distinct about the *third* week; is then about two lines long, weighing one to two grains; is surrounded by an amnion which lies loosely about it, and obviously proceeds from the abdominal laminæ; it presents cerebral vesicles; there is the appearance of an eye, several arteries are seen though not distinctly formed; the abdominal cavity is open for a considerable extent in front.

About the *fifth* week the embryo becomes more consistent; the head is disproportionately large; rudimentary eyes are indicated by two black spots; the abdomen is nearly closed, though at the umbilical aperture a loop of intestine escapes; the abdominal members are present, and the cord exists in a rudimentary condition; the embryo is nearly two-thirds of an inch long and weighs about fifteen grains.

The successive changes in the development were, 1st, a germ membrane visible immediately after the bursting of the vesicle; 2d, at some point an aggregation of granules forming the cumulus of the blastoderma; 3d, the embryo developed lying at this point, as it were upon the membranes, which consist of three superimposed laminæ or layers; 4th, on the serous layer arise the organs of animal life, the brain and spinal marrow, organs of sense, skin, muscles, tendons, ligaments, cartilage, and bone; on the mucous the organs of vegetative life, the intestinal canal, lungs, liver, spleen, pancreas and other glands. The heart and vascular system arise from the vascular layer (if this can be considered a separate one).

About the second week, or perhaps the third, there is a mass of globules loosely connected together forming the *primitive streak of Von Baer,* and around this the *area vasculosa* is developed. The globules of the primitive streak, seem next to be developed into two laminæ dorsales, which is the axis of the future embryo, and the origin of the spinal column. That portion of the fluid that separates the *chorda dorsalis* from the lamina dorsalis is the future spinal cord, and brain. Two other lamina—*laminæ ventrales of Von Baer*—are in the mean time proceeding from the axis of the embryo, one on each side; they grow laterally and converge below the axis.

After the rudiments of organic life have been commenced in the central portion of the serous layer, a fold of its peripheral portion arches over the dorsal surface of the embryo so as to represent a sac, and is composed of two membranes; the one next to the fœtus is the *amnion*, the other is gradually separated from the amnion and joins the serous lamina of the blastoderma; this is the *false amnion* of Pander.

The heart is formed at this early period, and although there is no septum between the ventricles, a vein may be seen entering into it, and an artery passes out which divides into four branches to be distributed and ramified in different portions of the fœtus.

The abdomen is yet an open cleft, in which (but projecting beyond it) is the heart, which is of very large dimensions; behind the heart is the liver, and under the liver the intestine which is attached by means of a distinct mesentery. At this period (three weeks) the lungs are constituted of five or six lobules, and two large glandular structures may also be discerned along the vertebral column, which are called Wolfian bodies; these anticipate the function of the kidneys. The *alantois* is seen arising from the lower part of the intestinal canal on a little vesicle and extending so as to encircle the embryo.

During the second month the extremities are growing, and become more projecting; the body is curved and the head bent downwards; there are indications of the nostrils and a gaping oral aperture; the forehead is more swelled because of the development of the hemispheres of the brain; the spinal cord is cylindrical of nearly uniform thickness and terminating in a blunt extremity—posteriorly it is open; the *medulla oblongata* makes a bend forwards at the top of the neck, and then ascends perpendicularly into the capacious cranium.

The first centres of ossification appear about the seventh week on the clavicle and lower jaw. At this time the kidneys and renal capsules begin to appear. The only trace of muscular fibre is in the diaphragm. The vertebral arches are not yet closed in, and the ribs appear like little streaks; the liver is very large and granular. The stomach is assuming somewhat of its normal form; the urinary bladder is enclosed, but the anus is imperforate. At this time the embryo is about an inch in length.

At two months the rudimentary organs of generation may be distinguished, but their development does not clearly show the sex. The embryo is from one and a half to two inches long and weighs near half an ounce, the head forming two-thirds of the whole.

After this period the different parts are developed with tolerable rapidity. At *ten weeks* the embryo is about two and a half inches in length. At the end of the *third month* it is from five to six inches long and weighs from three to four ounces. The thorax is closed at all points but is only slightly developed; the cord contains no intestines, and its spiral turns are evident; the nails are beginning to appear; the sex is distinct, and the skin acquires some consistence. At the fourth month the fœtus is six to eight inches in length, and weighs from seven to eight ounces. A fœtus born at this period might live for an hour or two. At *five months* the length of the body, including head and feet, is from eight to ten inches, and weighs from eight to eleven ounces; at *six months* the weight is about one pound, and the length is eleven to twelve and a half inches.

At *seven months* the fœtus is from twelve and a half to fourteen inches long and weighs from three to five pounds. The hands and feet, including the nails, are developed; all its parts are tolerably firm, and their respective dimensions better proportioned than formerly. The scrotum usually contains one or both testicles, they having descended through the inguinal ring, from their original place near the vertebral column; the eyelids are partly open; the skin is very red and covered with down. Many children live and are reared that are born at seven months.

The length of a fœtus born at term is eighteen or nineteen inches, though the utmost limit is more than two feet. The usual weight is from six to seven pounds; children have been born, however, that were as much as eighteen pounds in weight. I suspect that this will never occur unless the term has been extended beyond the usual period.

At term the fœtus that is twenty inches long will generally measure ten and a half to eleven inches from the crown to the umbilicus. The different parts are well developed and partly covered by a smegma called the *vernix caseosa*; the head has attained the proper hardness, and the scrotum usually contain the testicles. In female children the nymphæ are generally covered entirely by the labia, the breasts project, and in both sexes contain frequently a milky fluid.

As soon as the child that has been carried the full time is born it usually cries, opens its eyes, and makes some struggling motions with its limbs; it soon passes urine and feces, and readily takes the breast.

With occasional exceptions the position of the child is unaltered from an early period of pregnancy to its termination, whether the head be upwards or downwards. The arms are generally folded over the chest, the knees drawn up to the abdomen; the back curved, and the head bent upon the chest, so as to occupy as little space as possible. In ordinary cases the head is directed downwards, and the face looks obliquely, so that in the first and second position the back of the fœtus is turned partly forwards, and the belly in the third and fourth. We are enabled in many cases to ascertain the position of the fœtus in the uterus before labor has commenced, by means of the stethescope, by noting whether the pulsation is felt on one side or the other of the abdomen and observing whether it is heard clearly or not.

The longitudinal diameter of the head is from 4 to 4½ inches, the transverse from 3½ to 4, the vertical 3 to 3¾ inches. The transverse diameter of the shoulders and thorax is 4¾ to 5½; the widest diameter of the hips 4 to 5 inches. In general the measurements are a little less in the female than in the male.

The head of the fœtus is large, and as it is less compressible at term than other portions it merits a particular description; we should be acquainted with all its characters, that we may recognize them and thereby determine the position during labor.

The fœtal head is ovoidal in form, the large extremity being posterior. Several bones enter into the formation of the cranium; they are, 1st, the *frontal* bone forming the forehead; in the fœtus even at term it is usually divided; 2d, the two *parietal* bones, one on each side of the head, meeting on the median line at the top of the head; they help to form the vault of the cranium; 3d, the occipital bone, forming the posterior and part of the base of the skull; and 4th, the temporal bones, one on the right and one on the left side below the parietal, completing the lateral portions of the cranium and contributing to form the base of it. The cranial bones are not united to each other by sutures as they are in the adult, but are separated, the parietal bones especially, by membranous intervals, the intervals being larger in some children than in others. These intervals, or *sutures* and *fontanelles*, must be carefully studied.

The *sagittal suture* is the antero-posterior one, and extends from the root of the nose to the occipital bone. It is formed in front by the interval that separates the frontal bone into two halves, and superiorly by that between the two parietals. There is a suture which crosses this, called the transverse or *coronal suture*, which is formed by the space existing between the frontal and parietal bones. When the sagittal suture arrives at the superior angle of the occipital bone, it seems to part and give rise to two oblique lateral sutures which are called *lambdoidal*; these are formed by the posterior borders of the parietal bones and the superior one of the occipital.

Just at the point where the coronal and the lambdoidal sutures join the sagittal one, two membranous spaces, larger than those just described, are found; these have received the name of *fontanelles*.

In cases of head presentation during labor, one or the other of the fontanelles may be felt by the attending practitioner, and this indicates to him the position of the head and the presentation.

The *anterior fontanelle* presents an extensive surface at the place where the transverse crosses the sagittal suture. It is lozenge-shaped, and is bounded by four bony angles.

The *posterior fontanelle* is formed by the union of the two lambdoidal sutures with the termination of the sagittal suture. It is smaller than the anterior one, and is of a triangular form. It is bounded by the occipital bone and the angles of the parietal bones. During labor the bones may overlap each other so that the sutures cannot be felt, but the prominences of the bony margins will aid the diagnosis.

THE PHYSIOLOGY OF FŒTAL LIFE.

The ovule, after it arrives in the uterine cavity, comes in contact at all points with the mucous membrane of the uterus. Its nutrition at first is organic by superficial imbibition; afterwards, probably the villi of the chorion imbibe the fluids there secreted, and transmit them into the space between the chorion and the amnion, thence it transcends through the walls of the amnion, and a portion is conveyed into the fœtus through the umbilical vesicle. After the placenta is formed there may still be some absorption of some of the nutritive matters contained in the liquor amnii through the skin of the fœtus, but its growth is principally maintained by an assimilation of that which the radicles of the umbilical vessels take up in the placenta. By means of the extensive contact existing between the vascular apparatus of the two placentas, a transudation probably takes place of some part of the maternal blood, which is absorbed and mingled with the fœtal blood, and furnishes some of the nutritive material.

When mingled with the fœtal blood, the nutritive elements supplied by the mother are devoted to the development of the organs. It is supposed, however, that they undergo changes in the large liver of the fœtus and in its intestines.

There is no true respiration in the uterine cavity, but one function of the placenta is to renew the blood of the fœtus from that of the mother, in about the same way that the blood of fishes is ærated by the water passing through the gills.

Whether in the earlier months absorption is carried on by the surface alone, or whether a portion of the liquor amnii finds its way to the stomach is difficult to decide, but, without doubt, a certain amount of digestion is carried on.

The CIRCULATION of the blood in the fœtus cannot be understood without referring to certain anatomical peculiarities that do not exist in the adult. These characteristics depend on the absence of respiration, and disappear when it is established.

1st. The septum between the auricles of the heart is imperfect, having in its center a valvular oval aperture called the *foramen ovale.*

2d. The pulmonary artery, soon after its origin, gives off a branch, the *ductus arteriosis,* which enters the aorta just below the arch. The pulmonary arteries are very small.

3d. The *umbilical artery* in the *fœtus* is a large vascular trunk, which is nearly obliterated in after life. The two umbilical arteries run forwards and inwards along the lateral and superior parts of the bladder, then curve forwards to the abdominal wall, along which they ascend to the umbilicus, then pass along the cord to the placenta.

4th. The fœtus further differs from the adult in having an umbilical vein, which comes from the placental tissue, traverses the length of the cord, passes through the umbilical ring, is mostly distributed to the liver, but has a supplemental vein situated at the thick edge of the liver, and leading to the vena cava ascendens, called the *ductus venosis.*

The general effect of all these peculiarities is to render the heart virtually a single one; to provide for the quiescent state of the lungs, and to modify the distribution of fresh blood.

THE COURSE OF THE BLOOD IN THE FŒTUS IS AS FOLLOWS: The blood circulating in the umbilical vein is, on entering the fœtus, a part of it discharged through the *ductus venosis* into the vena cava; another part is distributed to the liver, and is brought to the vena cava by the hepatic veins, and then mingles also with that from the inferior extremities, and then with that from the upper extremities as it passes into the right auricle. A part of this is transmitted through the right ventricle, and thence (except a supply for the nourishment of the lungs) through the ductus arteriosis into the descending aorta. A second and larger part passes through the foramen ovale into the left auricle, then into the left ventricle and arch of the aorta, the branches of which supply the head and upper extremities. The continued stream passes into the descending aorta, mixing with that already described. The whole now descends to the lower part of the aorta, where a portion is sent to the inferior extremities, but a larger part is drawn into the umbilical arteries, and is carried by them into the placenta.

After birth remarkable changes take place. Something in the circumstances in which the child is placed stimulates respiration and crying, by which means the lungs are inflated, and space is afforded to the pulmonary circulation, which supercedes the use of the foramen ovale and ductus arteriosis; the blood from the lower extremities cannot pass through the umbilical arteries, and does pass through the ascending cava into the right auricle and ventricle, then into the lungs, where it undergoes analagous changes to those effected in the placenta, and is distributed to the body generally. The fœtal openings are generally obliterated in the course of a week, though the foramen ovale, or the ductus venosis, may continue pervious for two or three weeks; but soon the ductus venosis and the umbilical arteries are obliterated and the adult circulation established.

CHAPTER I.
DIAGNOSIS OF PREGNANCY.

A few of the early signs of pregnancy are not made available to the physician ordinarily when his opinion is demanded. A woman is naturally unwilling that her physician, if he be a man, should make even a digital examination, and this makes it more necessary that the nurse should know all the rational signs.

One of these signs is the changed color of the mucous membrane of the vagina and labia. This membrane is of a pale red color, but it becomes of a violet hue during the time of menstruation, and if a woman becomes pregnant, the violet or deep red color becomes continuous.

There is also, even in the commencement of pregnancy, a peculiar odor to the secretion from the vagina and os uteri, which has been compared to that of the vernix caseosa.

There is no sign of pregnancy by which we can always distinguish it in its early stages; in some instances nearly all the rational signs are absent. The general condition of a pregnant woman is changed in a greater or less degree, but all are not changed alike.

Generally she is plethoric, the pulse is fuller and quicker; the quantity of circulating fluid is augmented, the quality altered by the increase of fibrine; but these changes are not always obvious. Well marked sympathies are excited in various organs; the nervous system may suffer especially; the woman's temper and disposition may change; she may become capricious, may have likes and dislikes in eating, especially if her digestion is weak; there may be loss of appetite, heartburn, increased flow of saliva, toothache, excitability of mind, sleepiness, etc.; but even when many of these symptoms are present, even when the liver and kidneys are affected, so that the skin is sallow or discolored in patches, and irritability of the bladder causes much pain and distress, these various signs may only furnish a sum of probabilities amounting *almost* to certainty.

In some cases of pregnancy the skin, instead of becoming sallow, is more florid, with occasional eruptions on the face.

Some women become fat during pregnancy; others lose flesh; their faces, in the early months, are pinched and pointed, and their features altered.

Milk in the breasts, especially in the first pregnancy, is a sign which is said to be reliable; but it is true of some women that, during their period of menstruation, their breasts enlarge; there is a sensation of fullness, with throbbing and tingling pain in them, and that a milk fluid may be secreted; the same symptoms that are present with others at the second month of pregnancy.

Another change is a more marked sign in the breasts. There is at first a soft and moist state of the skin, and the little glandular follicles around the nipples are bedewed with a secretion. This may often be seen at the second month, and it may also be noticed that the veins of the breast look more blue, and that the breasts themselves are firmer and more knotty to the touch.

There are, however, other signs which are more to be depended on than these that have been mentioned.

Females *cease to be regular during pregnancy*. A healthy married woman, during the period of child-bearing, bases her prediction upon this sign, and is seldom disappointed. But women are not all healthy; disease and disorder of the womb, or other organs of the body, especially of the lungs, may cause suppression of the catamenia; and, on the other hand, the discharge may recur for several months after conception, or even monthly during the period of utero gestation; and, in anomalous cases, some young married women, who had hitherto been quite regular, ceased to menstruate for several months without any known cause.

Morning sickness is one of the earliest signs of pregnancy, as it often occurs within two weeks. The nausea may be slight or it may be very distressing; it may happen to be soon relieved, but it usually continues for three or four months or longer. It varies also as regards the time of day during which it continues to be bad; but if it recurs at the regular time and in the regular manner, it is of great value as an evidence of pregnancy, when combined with other symptoms.

A dark brown areola around the nipple may usually be noticed at the end of the second month; this is a distinguishing sign, especially if it be a first pregnancy. A month or two later, the dark color is more obvious, and it is darker in persons with dark hair, etc. It may be described as being a dark circle, somewhat swollen, or with a puffy turgescence, both of the nipple and the surrounding disk; the surface of the areola studded over and rendered unequal by the prominence of the glandular follicles, the integument covering the part soft and moist; sometimes small mottled patches, of a whitish color, scattered over the outer surface of the areola, and for about an inch all around it.

These marks are quite plain at the fifth month, and at six months a number of silvery *streaks* may be observed.

Quickening is one of the most important signs of pregnancy, and occurs about the fourth or fifth month; not because the child is then first alive, but because the womb then rises higher in the abdomen, and because the child has reached a further state of development. Quickening is a proof that the woman is near half her time gone; though it may happen that the sensation is observed as early as the third or fourth month, instead of at four and a half months. In some cases women do not know the time when they quicken, as only a slight sensation is felt; this some compare to the fluttering of a bird. But a lady may at that time be faint, or giddy, or sick, though there seemed to be nothing more than a mere pulsation. Subsequently, however, the movements become stronger and more frequent. The motions of the child may be felt by a third person on placing the hand on the woman's abdomen, especially if the person's hand be cold. I have known one case in which, by placing my hand on the woman's abdomen, I caused motions which simulated active movements of the child, although there was no fœtus present.

INCREASED SIZE AND HARDNESS OF THE ABDOMEN is characteristic of pregnancy. Enlargement of the abdomen may be from flatulence, but such enlargement is not persistent; the belly is large one hour and small the next, and on pressing the bowels firmly, a rumbling of wind may be heard, which perhaps may move about, and on percussing (tapping) the part, a hollow sound may be elicited, as from a drum. A large abdomen may be due to fat, but there is a soft and doughy feeling that is characteristic of fat. On the contrary, in pregnancy, hardness, solidity and resistance to pressure characterize the gravid uterus, and the enlargement is not only persistent, but gradually increasing. It is true that when a very fat woman is pregnant, percussion or palpation of the abdomen may be fruitless, and any certain diagnosis cannot be made, but in most cases, if we are careful to observe these conditions, and also whether there is a distended bladder and rectum, the diagnosis can be made after the fourth or fifth month.

To make an examination by percussion and palpation, let the female lie down, with the head raised and the thighs flexed on the abdomen; then examine with both hands, especially near the pubis. Pressure with the ends of all the fingers, gradually moving them upward, will enable us to detect the womb, if it rise above the symphasis, and also the size and height of the fundus.

Ballottement, or *repercussion,* is used as a means of deciding upon the presence of a fœtus; a means that is most available about the fifth and sixth month. The female examined should be in an upright position, or if she be in bed, her shoulders should be raised. We are directed to introduce the forefinger into the vagina and touch the cervix uteri, or, rather, in front of the neck upon the walls of the uterus; then slightly jerking upward by slightly flexing the first joint of the finger; observe if something recede from it and fall again in a moment. The ballottement is said to be a sensation "analagous to that produced by placing a ball of marble in a bladder full of water and then striking the bladder with the finger just under where the ball rests, when the latter is thrown up and falls from its own weight upon the finger that displaced it."

When the vaginal touch is practiced, while one finger remains in the vagina, palpation of the uterus with the other hand may assist in the diagnosis by depressing the uterus, or by holding it firmly in place. Then the jerk of the finger upon the head of the fœtus causes it to float upwards a little in the liquor amnii and descend.

AUSCULTATION is used to decide many cases of doubtful pregnancy. The pulsations of the fœtal heart are generally perceptible by the fifth month. The examination may be made by applying the naked ear to the abdomen of the mother, she being placed on her back in the bed with her head raised.

The *fœtal pulsations* are frequent, generally from 120 to 140 a minute. The *uterine souffle* or bellows murmur may often be heard as early as the fourth month; it is synchronous with the mother's pulse; its seat is said to be the uterus, and some believe that it indicates the position of the placenta. This sound and the *pulsation of the umbilical cord* are not very important diagnostic signs, and the same may be said of the presence of *kiestiene* in the urine, which may, however, be detected as early as the third month.

Some of the ailments that attend pregnancy I will now merely mention: There may be irritability and a disposition to inflammation; violent and obstinate vomiting; indigestion and depraved appetite, heartburn, costiveness, hemorrhoids, liver spots or blotches, especially about the face; diarrhœa or dysentery; strangury, with a frequent inclination to void the urine; leucorrhœa; varicose veins in the legs, thigh and abdomen; inquietude, and sleeplessness; dropsy, or an œdematous condition of the lower extremities; prurigo vulva; either of these may be more or less troublesome, but can hardly be regarded as diagnostic signs. Some remedies for these will be mentioned hereafter. (F. 69, 72, 75, 81, 131, 173, 206, 220).

The abdominal walls are often distended beyond what the woman is able to bear without inconvenience, as the skin may become inflamed and crack. It is much more common that the true skin beneath the epidermis cracks, and, although the outside is not altered, there often remains upon the abdomen of women who have had children a number of small marks, or little whitish streaks.

CHAPTER II.
ABORTION.

If a premature expulsion of the fœtus occur before the end of the seventh month, it is called an *abortion, or miscarriage*; subsequent to this period, premature labor.

The cause of abortion may be in the ovum or in the mother, and it is more liable to occur at the beginning of each month corresponding to the menstrual period. The maternal causes may arise from the condition of the mother or may be accidental; may be anything that injuriously affects the mind or body. Debility of constitution, consumption, leucorrhœa, uterine irritation, febrile complaints, and obstinate constipation may be causes, but some women who are weak or sick retain the ovum with wonderful tenacity. Blows, falls, violent concussions, excessive or sudden exertions, straining, severe coughing, taking long walks, riding on horseback, or over rough roads in a carriage, a long railway journey, fright, sudden shocks, anger, joy, sorrow, good or bad news suddenly told, taking a wrong step in ascending or descending stairs, lifting heavy weights, violent drastic purgatives, calomel, dancing, and tight lacing may excite the uterus to action and effect the expulsion of its contents.

It is an unfortunate thing for a woman if she miscarry with her first and second child, for it often becomes a habit. Having once miscarried, she is more likely to miscarry again, and by repeated miscarriages her constitution is broken, and the chances of her ever having a living child become very small.

A woman may experience some *threatening or warning symptoms of miscarriage* for one or two days before those of labor supervene. There is usually a feeling of languor or weariness, of lassitude and depression of spirits, and a sense of uneasiness, and then, after these premonitory symptoms have lasted for some time, there may be a discharge of mucus or blood from the vagina. The show may increase to flooding, and soon there may be pain, at first slight and irregular, afterwards of a grinding character, and subsequently severe, irregular, and bearing down. At this stage we may be quite certain that the pains will continue to recur until the fœtus at least, if not the afterbirth, have passed into the vagina.

The progress in different cases is, however, quite dissimilar. In the beginning of pregnancy the expulsion of the ovum might closely follow the accident that caused it. For example, a woman might slip in descending a staircase and fall violently on her seat, causing immediate expulsion of the ovum, with a large quantity of fluid blood. There are some women who have acquired the habit of aborting, and the ovum passes out of the womb with scarcely any pain, little or no hemorrhage, and the woman speedily recovers. But it will very seldom happen, after the first six weeks, that there is not some interval between the accident and the consequent abortion, and that there is not considerable and protracted pain.

If the cause of the abortion affects the mother instead of the ovum, she generally experiences, at the time of the accident, a sharp pain about the loins or abdomen, which may continue slightly for several days, and then be renewed, with violent uterine contractions, and some serous and then bloody discharges from the vagina.

The progress of a miscarriage is not as regular as a labor at full term. In many cases there are shiverings succeeded by fever for a day or more preceding the hemorrhage. Severe indisposition may continue for several days. There may be not only considerable uterine pain, but much pain in the bladder and loins; a sense of sinking in the epigastrium, of weight near the vulva and anus, and an ineffectual desire to urinate.

Such symptoms continue a longer or shorter time, and then usually the fœtus alone is expelled, the placenta being retained. The latter is generally detached after a time, or it may (if within the first three months) be discharged and pass out in a dissolved condition, with the lochia. Very alarming hemorrhage may precede and accompany abortion; this makes the case one of danger at the time, and may permanently affect the health of the woman afterwards. The flooding may continue after the expulsion of the ovum; but I have always found that in such cases there was a portion of the placenta that was detached, and that might be removed, though not perhaps without some difficulty. A good physician should always be called in cases of continued flooding.

The patient ought always to preserve any and every substance discharged, that it may be showed to the physician. He should make a digital examination, and he usually finds the os uteri to be partially dilated, and a portion of the placenta hanging in the orifice. It has always been my practice to see that all was removed before leaving my patient, and I have known very dangerous hemorrhage to occur where this rule was not observed. The placenta can generally be seized by two fingers and removed; but if persevering efforts are necessary, they should not be relinquished until the safety of the mother is assured, which cannot be while the ovum, or membranes, or placenta remain in the uterus separated from their connections.

But it should always be considered especially important to PREVENT THE ABORTION. If a woman is prone to miscarry, she ought, as soon as she is pregnant, to lie down a great part of the day; she must keep her mind calm and unruffled, and must live on plain diet; she should retire early to rest, and *she must have a separate sleeping apartment*. She should avoid taking active physic, but keep her bowels open by diet or by the mildest aperients, or, possibly, daily enemata. Gentle exercise may be taken, alternated with frequent rest. Cold ablutions are proper every morning, but the body should be rubbed afterwards with a coarse towel.

The most usual time for a woman to miscarry is from the eighth to the thirteenth week, but if a woman have a particular time, which to her is the usual period, whenever that time approaches she should be unusually careful. Let her lie down more than she usually does; let her avoid exciting amusements. She might try to keep her bowels open by the external application of castor oil, or by the mildest aperients, or by hot water enemata.

If slight hemorrhage and trifling pains come on, we should seek to arrest the abortion by giving perhaps grain doses of opium every four or five hours. If the hemorrhage is severe, a drachm dose of fluid extract of ergot may be given, and a large draught of cinnamon tea; perhaps a quarter of a grated nutmeg, and, in extreme cases, a spoonful of brandy with it.

But let it be understood that in all such cases a physician should be called as soon as possible; and while waiting for him the patient ought to lie on a hair mattress; a vaginal injection of hot water may be given; she should have but scant clothing upon the bed; her room should be well ventilated, and if she is faint from the loss of blood, a little aromatic ammonia may be given.

CHAPTER III.
PARTURITION.

FALSE PAINS occur most frequently in a first pregnancy, but most pregnant women have occasional pains, and these become more violent within three weeks of the full time. They may be owing to a disordered stomach, as well as to the action of the uterus; but they usually come on at night, and are liable to be mistaken for labor pains. They are, however, unattended with show; they often change from place to place, perhaps going successively to the hips, loins, lower extremities and abdomen; they come on at irregular intervals, and are at one time violent, at another feeble, and they occasion no dilation of the os uteri; but true pains come on with some regularity, and usually increase in severity. False pains are from various causes, such as fatigue of any kind, especially too long standing, sudden and violent motions of the body, costiveness or diarrhœa, general feverishness, agitation of the mind, or a spasmodic action of the abdominal muscles. It is necessary to adopt the means used for the relief of the pains to the apparent cause, and generally to give an opiate proportioned to the degree of pain, or to repeat in small quantities at proper intervals till the patient shall be composed.

PERIOD OF GESTATION.

The duration of pregnancy is not always absolutely a certain number of days. The usual term is ten lunar months, or nine calendar months and one week. If we could have correct records of all cases we should probably find that half the cases of pregnancy terminated in labor in the fortieth week, but that in a few instances the term was prolonged to the forty-fifth week and that in as many cases women were delivered of fully developed children as early as the thirty-seventh week.

A woman may make her count pretty correctly as follows: She should first note the last day of her being unwell. Let forty weeks from that day be marked in an almanac, and she may expect her labor to come on near that time.

It may happen that a woman who never has her menses while she is suckling, may become pregnant and not have a date to count from; but she ought in that case to reckon from the time that she quickens. Although quickening takes place at various periods, she may then consider herself nearly half gone in her pregnancy, and calculate that in four and a half months she will be delivered.

A woman may have a show for one or two monthly periods after her gestation commences, but the discharge may be distinguished from the regular menstrual fluid by its being either small in quantity, or by its clotting, and generally by its lasting but a few hours. The woman should reckon from the time when she had her last regular menstruation.

PARTURITION.

NATURAL LABOR. The uterine functions are characterized by periodicity. If an abortion occurs that is not the result of an accident, it is generally at what would have been, but for conception, a monthly period, and even injuries are more likely to produce their bad effects at that particular time. So the normal period for parturition corresponds to a menstrual period, and generally labor may be looked for at about the tenth period after the last appearance of the catamenia. We can hardly tell why it so uniformly happens at that particular time; the process is analagous to the falling of ripe fruit—it drops because the fruit is fully matured.

It is not in accordance with the plan of this work to dwell at all upon any other than what is called natural labor, but I shall include in this class all such as are terminated by the natural powers, whether they be head, face, breach, or foot presentations.

By PRESENTATION, I mean that part that presents itself at the brim of the pelvis, so that the accoucheur's finger impinges upon it as the end is passed into the center of the os uteri.

The DIAGNOSIS of the different presentations is made by the touch. The head may be known by the hardness and roundness, and more certainly by the fontanelles and sutures; the breach by its general softness, and by the tuberosity of the haunch bone; by the cleft between the buttocks, the scrotum or the vulva, and the anus; the knee by the hardness and roundness of the bone; the foot by its form, its being at right angles with the leg, the nearly equal length of the toes, the narrow heel, etc.; and the face by the inequalities of the presenting part. (These inequalities cannot at first be felt; upon touching it we first perhaps detect the brow, then, as labor progresses, we may feel the nose, mouth, etc.) The head presents in about 98 cases out of 100.

PHYSIOLOGICAL PHENOMENA OF LABOR.

According to the division made by standard authors on parturition, its first stage extends from the beginning of labor to the complete dilatation of the os uteri; the second terminates by the birth of the child, and the third by the expulsion of the placenta.

During the last two or three weeks of the term, the uterus sinks lower in the pelvis, and seems to spread out laterally; the lungs and stomach are not so much compressed, and respiration and digestion, if difficult, become more easy, and often the patient becomes more cheerful and active. The precursory symptoms of labor vary in intensity in different women; but it may be observed pretty generally that there is more activity and disposition to movement for one day preceding the real labor.

But during the last few days of the gestation there are contractions of the uterus, which, though short and distant, and not attended with much pain, are effective in dilating the cervix, and preparing for the subsequent labors.

The subsidence of the lower end of the uterus into the pelvis, however, causes many unpleasant symptoms. The pressure upon the bladder renders a frequent evacuation of its contents necessary; there is often an ineffectual desire to urinate, and sometimes strangury. There is often a sense of weight about the anus, an irritable state of the bowels, occasional griping pains, and a desire to go to stool when but little is passed, and sometimes diarrhœa. The œdema and varices of the lower extremities augment, the hemorrhoidal vessels swell up, and the piles are larger. These precursory symptoms are manifested more in primapara than in others. To some, walking becomes at this time impossible.

There are during the last month, and especially toward the close of it, painless uterine contractions; there may be at first a sort of squeezing sensation with it. But about twenty-four hours previous to the commencement of actual labor, these contractions are accompanied with some pain and are periodical, recurring perhaps every twenty or thirty minutes. If an examination be made of the os tincæ at the COMMENCEMENT OF LABOR it will be found that the rounded collar of the os is already effaced. The pains then suddenly become acute, and it can be observed that the uterus contracts if we notice its greater hardness and roundness during a pain. The os uteri if somewhat dilated closes partially with each contracting, and it can be observed that its margins are growing thinner though tense and resistant at the time of the pain.

The contractions distend the membranes; these are first pressed *on* the neck, then *into* it, then as soon as the dilatation is sufficiently advanced engage in it in the form of the segment of a sphere, whose dimensions progressively increase with the dilatations.

There is now and perhaps has been for several hours a glairy discharge from the vagina, which becomes streaked with blood, there are perhaps shiverings or rigors (not accompanied with a cold skin), the pains increase in force and frequency, the pulse is hard, full, and rather frequent, the countenance is flushed, often there is vomiting, and the patient is prone to despond and be discouraged.

She is less agitated after the pain subsides, though it does not cease entirely. During the interval the margins of the os again become supple, the membrane that was tense while the pain lasted becomes flaccid, and the child's head can be more plainly felt. As the contractions are repeated the os uteri dilates more and more until it is completely opened and no part of its margin can be touched; though very frequently from some obliquity of the uterus, the margin on one side can be observed pushed down before the head of the child, while that on the other side cannot be reached. In ordinary cases the membranes are ruptured and the waters escape at the commencement of the second stage, and the time occupied by the first stage is nearly three-fourths that for the whole labor. But the duration of the stages as well as the time occupied by the parturition is exceedingly variable, and the same may be said in regard to the duration and character of the pain.

We may observe here that pain is nearly inseparable from the contractions of the uterus, so that in common language the two expressions are used indifferently; but using the word in its ordinary sense the pain in the first stage of labor is different from that in the second. What are called grinding pains characterize the first part of labor, and although they differ in different individuals, they are pretty generally so severe as to cause the patient to cry out. As soon as the labor advances to *the second stage* there is a change in the character of the pains. They are more frequent and longer and the intervals shorter; but though the suffering may be greater the cry is more suppressed, the bearing down is carried to a greater degree, and each pain is succeeded by a calm more perfect than that in the first stage. Should the interval be rather long some patients get a little sleep between the pains, but if there has not been a bursting of the waters previously there is generally now a pain sufficiently hard to break the membrane.

Either in the first or last part, or during the whole of the labor, the woman says that the pain is in her back, it being in the lumber and dorsal region; the grinding pain she speaks of as being forward, they seem however to go through from the umbilicus to the sacrum. In cases where there is rigidity of the uterine orifice, there is I believe pain especially in the back; and when the os becomes fully dilated, the pains are bearing down; the patient at the accession of a pain holds her breath, and seizing hold of something with her hands, brings the muscles of the back and abdomen and extremities to aid the expulsive efforts of the uterus. I do not doubt that this straining of the mother at this time is advantageous; these efforts of the mother should not be encouraged, however, at the first part of the labor, because then they do no good, nor at the very last, as combined efforts then may rupture the perineum.

As the head advances through the pelvic cavity the pressure upon the nerves which pass through it gives rise to cramps in the thighs and legs.

As the head passes into the vagina the walls become flabby and the canal seems to enlarge and elongate and to be prepared to yield to the pressure of the head. If an internal examination be made the head will be perceived filling the cavity, descending with each pain and receding at its conclusion—the advance ordinarily exceeding the recession, though sometimes the gain is not perceptible. When the head rests on the perineum, that offers some resistance, which seems to stimulate the uterus and abdominal muscles to greater efforts and more forcible contractions.

If it be a first labor there may be at this point a little delay in its progress. But the fœtal head being forced down by the rapidly recurring pains so presses against the floor of the pelvis that it yields and becomes bulging in front, and distended, though there still is recession as the pain intermits. But adequate force is called into action; each pain gains upon the advance made by its predecessor; the vulva partially opens, and at each pain they open more and more; the resistance of the parts is finally overcome. After the perineum has given the head its proper direction in its transit, there usually comes a hard pain—forcing a loud cry from the woman—another pain succeeds immediately, which expels the head altogether from the parts; then after a short rest the uterine power is again exerted to expel the body of the child.

There may be an interval of a few minutes before the pains return with sufficient force to expel the shoulders, but the child is in no particular danger; it is best to wait awhile, the nurse in the meantime making pressure with her hand over the uterus, before any traction is made on the head or shoulders. If the body is very large, however, it may be well soon to draw a little on the head or to reach with one finger into the axilla and to bring down the lower shoulders; then the rest will be delivered without any difficulty.

The intense suffering of the mother is now exchanged for perfect joy or ease; there is at once a transition from extreme misery to total freedom from pain, though the labor is not yet completed. Ordinarily a few pains return before many minutes, and complete the last stage of labor—the expulsion of the placenta. Sometimes the contractions that expel the child, expel also the membranes and placenta; but more generally they are only partially detached or they may be adherent and not easily removed.

After the birth of the child, and the tying of the naval string, it is proper to apply the hand upon the abdomen of the mother to ascertain whether there be another child, and whether the uterus be contracting properly. I advise that an effort should be made immediately to remove the afterbirth and secundines, making firm pressure over the womb; this will generally stimulate the uterus to make good contractions, and may assist in pressing out the placenta. I do not advise that a midwife should pull upon the cord, but it is my practice to press the fingers of my right hand well into the vagina, and as soon as possible grasp a little of the placenta; my left hand at the same time pulling slightly on the cord, and thus by combined effort removing the afterbirth pretty quickly.

I have never had much trouble about retained or adherent placenta in cases where I myself officiated in the delivery, and I attribute my good fortune in this respect to the fact that I do not tie the placental portion of the cord, preferring to let some blood discharge from the afterbirth, thus diminishing its size, and then if necessary I direct that considerable effort be made in the way of squeezing and pressure and friction over the uterus.

It is true that if nothing is done a pain will usually come on within twenty minutes that will expel the afterbirth very effectually including all the membranes, and considerable clots of blood; but I apprehend that in many cases during this delay there is an hour-glass contraction of the womb comes on, which retains the placenta and prevents its proper separation.

But before attending to the placenta, the necessary attention should be paid to the child. A little cold water sprinkled on it will usually make the child cry, if it does not breath immediately after it is born, and this makes the change in it from uterine to breathing life. The child may then be separated from the mother by cutting the cord. After the removal of the child it is proper to endeavor to deliver the afterbirth, though it may not be necessary at first to do anything more than to use friction over the uterus with moderate pressure, which may be gradually increased.

CHAPTER IV.
MECHANICAL PHENOMENA OF LABOR.

The cavity of the uterus and that of the pelvis form a continuous PASSAGE through which the child must be forced in its exit from the womb at birth. The uterus possesses the character of muscularity and is the main agent in the expulsion of the child. By its own muscular action the cavity of the uterus is diminished and pressure made on the fœtus, forcing it down towards the orifice, distending the cervix, and dilating the passage. During the second stage of labor the power of the uterus is aided by the voluntary muscles of the abdomen and by the depression of the diaphragm.

The character of the passage will be brought to mind by recalling what was heretofore said of the diameter of the pelvis. It will be remembered that the usual antero-posterior diameter of the brim does not exceed 4½ inches while the transverse is 5¼ inches, and that at the lower outlet the antero-posterior diameter is about 5 inches and the transverse about 4 inches.

The FIRST OBSTACLE which the child meets in its progress is the cervex uteri. This being composed partly of muscular fibre which acts somewhat as a sphincter, and partly of elastic celular tissue, holds the sphincter in the tissue with a tenacity which is not easily overcome. But repeated muscular contractions of the womb force down the bag of waters, which forms a sort of wedge, and this is forced down and into the os uteri, compelling it to open.

There are also muscular fibres in the uterus which have a longitudinal as well as some that have a circular course, and the action of the former tend after a time to retract the os, over the fœtal head.

The *second obstacle* is the bony brim of the pelvis into which the head of the fœtus cannot pass until its long diameter is adapted to certain diameters of the pelvis. The diameter of the bony pelvis is diminished over one-fourth of an inch by the soft parts upon it, but the oblique diameter of the pelvis will admit the long diameter of the head of the child, which does not often exceed 4½ inches. The head usually presents in this way, and passes in a somewhat spiral manner until it arrives at the outlet where the diameters are adjusted to each other. The head is, however, too large to pass, even in this way, were it not that it admits of a degree of compression to facilitate the entrance and progress through; this moulding is effected by the continued pains. The head of the child which presents at the brim with the occiput towards the left acetabulum rotates during the passage, so that the occiput at its exit is directly under the symphasis pubis; the cause of the rotation is found in the form and direction of the passage and in the shape and size of the fœtal head.

This presentation and position is the most common one, though either of the following is liable to occur. By naming the position we indicate just how a presenting part lies, or is turned. We adopt the following classification, which accords with several good authors:

PRESENTATIONS AND POSITIONS.

PRESENTATIONS.	No.	POSITION.	NAME OF POSITION.
	1	Occiput to left acetabulum.	Left occipito-iliac anterior.
	2	Occiput to right acetabulum.	Right occipito-iliac anterior.
	3	Occiput to Symphasis pubis.	Occipito pubic.
A—Vertex or head	4	Occiput to r. sacro-iliac junc.	R. occipito-iliac posterior.
	5	Occiput to l. sacro-iliac junc.	L. occipito-iliac posterior.
	6	Occiput to promon'y of sacrum	Occipito sacral.
	1	Sacrum to left acetabulum.	Left sacro-iliac anterior.
B—Breach, including inferior extremities.	2	Sacrum to right acetabulum.	Right sacro-iliac anterior.
	3	Sacrum to symphasis pubis.	Sacro pubic.
	4	Sacrum to r. sacro-iliac junction.	Left sacro-iliac posterior.
	5	Sacrum to l. sacro-iliac junction.	Right sacro-iliac posterior.
	6	Sacrum to promont'y of	Sacro sacral.

sacrum.

C—Body, including shoulders, elbow and hand.

D—Face, including six varieties.

The right occipito-iliac posterior (A 4) position is not a very uncommon one, but that variety which is described and named as the left occipito-iliac anterior (A 1), in which the occiput is directed in front and to the left, is most frequent. These and other vertex presentations may be recognized even in the commencement of labor through the vaginal walls, the head being known by its rounded spheroidal surface.

Supposing that we have a case of the kind that is most common (A 1), and that labor has begun, we may introduce the finger through the os uteri and we encounter a rounded, smooth and resistant surface, which is the anterior part of the head, and then by directing the finger upwards and backwards it will come in contact with the sagittal suture.

If the direction of the suture is oblique, and if it runs from before backwards and from the left towards the right, the position must be either the left anterior or the right posterior occipito-iliac one. (A 1 or A 4).

To complete the diagnosis we follow with the finger the sagittal suture until it reaches the fontanelle, and this determines the position. If the posterior fontanelle is found to the left and in front, and the anterior one is to the right and behind, the position is A 1, or the left antero-occipito-iliac one. The back of the fœtus is turned forwards and towards the left side, while its face and anterior plane is turned backwards and towards the right, and the occipito-frontal diameter of the child's head corresponds to the oblique diameter of the pelvic brim.

As the labor progresses and the head is forced down in the pelvis, it is also more strongly flexed on the chest and the occiput is pressed down in the excavation. With the occiput thus presenting, it traverses all the space between the superior and inferior straits until it reaches the floor of the pelvis; there it makes what is sometimes called the pivot turn—it executes a movement of rotation, which carries the occiput behind the symphasis pubis and the forehead towards the hollow of the sacrum; then the head being pressed forwards and stretching the perineum, the forehead and face being disengaged from it, emerge; then after the perfect expulsion of the head it again rotates, the occiput turns somewhat to the left thigh and the face towards the right thigh.

In the beginning of labor the shoulders are turned so as to correspond to the oblique diameter of the pelvic cavity, but they pass through the pelvis in a transverse position. After they reach the inferior strait, the body rotates so that the right shoulder of the child turns towards the left side of the mother and the wide diameter of the shoulders is accommodated to the wide diameter of the strait, and the rotation of the head, which is free externally, is secondary to the rotation of the shoulders.

In the EXPULSION OF THE BODY the right shoulder, or subpubic one, is the first one to appear in the vulvar fissure, but the left or posterior one may be disengaged at the commissure of the perineum before the right one is delivered; the remainder of the trunk is expelled very soon, describing a prolonged spiral course in its passage.

A child originally in the RIGHT POSTERIOR-ILIAC position becomes converted towards the last of the labor into an occipito pubic or anterior one, and the labor terminates as it does in A 1, when the occiput was originally in front. It is the left shoulder, however, which gets behind the arch of the pubis, and the occiput is directed towards the *right* thigh after the head emerges.

In some instances, though rarely, the child originally in A 4 position remains with the occiput behind to the termination of the labor. In such cases the forehead comes under the pubis and remains there for a time, while the occiput traverses the whole circle of the perineum; then the whole head and face is immediately delivered.

It is not deemed necessary to describe here the mechanism of labor in the more unusual varieties which are so very numerous.

As regards PROGNOSIS, head presentations are the most favorable of all, and those in which the occiput looks anteriorly in the beginning of labor are more favorable than those in which it is turned posteriorly. In occipito-posterior positions the labor is more tedious than when the occiput is in front, and the expulsion becomes particularly difficult when the head maintains its original position and does not rotate or take the pivot turn.

Upon the fœtal head after it is delivered there is almost always a protuberance to be found—a tumefaction, more or less considerable upon some point of the vertex; its greater size indicating a longer continuance of the labor, and its seat indicating in what position the child was born. This tumor is almost always located on one of the posterior superior angles of the parietal bones, and shows that the occiput escaped under the pubic arch.

During the labor the whole head is strongly compressed except at one point on the vertex, which therefore becomes the seat of a sero-sanguinolent infiltration. This tumor disappears usually within forty-eight hours; if it does not, it may properly be punctured. It may contain either serum, or serum and blood, or grumous blood.

CHAPTER V.
DIAGNOSIS OF ARTIFICIAL LABOR.

When the expulsion of the fœtus takes place from the efforts of nature alone, the labor is called by some authors spontaneous or natural, but when art is obliged to interfere it is called artificial. It would be very useful to us if we could always decide in the commencement of labor whether the assistance of art would be required, and I will group together in a few pages such instructions as I am able to give on this important subject.

The nurse or midwife will not very generally be able to decide any point by auscultation, but she as well as the physician may judge from the appearance of the woman, from her past history, from palpation of the abdomen, and from vaginal touch. She should accustom herself to judging by all these means, that she may be able to decide early whether the help of an accoucheur will be *imperatively* needed.

No one can decide certainly from simply seeing a patient in the beginning of labor, whether her labor will be natural and spontaneous, or artificial; but I have many times when first looking at a lady, if her complexion was fair, and her form good, but rather tall, predicted that her accouchement would proceed regularly and favorably. But in forming our opinion we need to know something of the previous health and present ailments of the patient, and, if a multipara, the character of former labors. If nausea and vomiting or any other ailment has reduced her strength so that she is exceedingly weak, this may give rise to some reasonable apprehension; but I have known a woman that could scarcely retain a morsel of food on her stomach for seven or eight months, that had become very weak indeed and exceedingly emaciated, who yet endured her labor well and soon recovered. The general rule is, that the more perfect the woman's health is, the better she is fitted for child bearing, but if her general health and strength is reduced below its proper standard by some previous or accompanying disease, such for example as consumption, she may endure the labor very well, and succumb to the disease afterwards.

Pregnant women are liable to be attacked with epidemic, endemic, and sporadic diseases. Eruptive fevers, etc., may attack parturient women, and if they do, the disease and labor in every case will have a reciprocal influence on each other—the disease will complicate the case. Influenza or intermittent fever may attack a woman at any period of gestation, and there may be no serious results. Cholera, small pox, typhoid fever, scarlet fever, measles, pneumonia, and jaundice are liable to cause abortion, and there is danger of fatal results, or either of them would be a dangerous complication at the time of labor. Syphilis would be a cause of abortion or premature labor, and any disease which allows the mother to carry the child the full term may reduce and weaken her. Glandular engorgements and scrofulous ulcers improve during gestation, but if the woman is suffering from a fracture, the bones will not unite very well. Tumors in the abdomen and pelvis may be an obstacle to delivery, and ulcerations of the cervix may also be harmful and protract the labor, as also may constipation, dropsy, and albuminuria.

The latter may not be detected without an analysis of the urine, but dropsy will be obvious as soon as it exists. The evidences of tumors and ulcerations are found by palpation and the touch—sometimes by the use of the speculum.

After learning the present appearance and the former history of the patient it may be necessary to examine further perhaps by palpation.

By PALPATION we may sometimes (but not always) distinguish the head of the child, and perhaps tell to which side its back is turned. When making the examination let the patient lie on her back, make gentle pressure when the pains are off and the abdomen is relaxed; press the ends of your fingers above the body of the pubis; by pressing downwards you may perhaps feel the head if it has descended into the pelvis. You will need to press the abdomen carefully all over to ascertain if there are tumors, and also to ascertain if the body or some other part presents at the cervix uteri.

If *auscultation* is used we may determine positively the position of the fœtus by observing just where the sounds of the fœtal heart may be most plainly heard.

The VAGINAL TOUCH is the usual mode of determining whether there is an unfavorable presentation of the child, as well as whether there is deformity of the pelvis, tumors in the vagina, ulcerations, &c.

When the head presents in the commencement of labor, if the fundus of the uterus is not too much inclined forwards, and there is no deformity of the pelvis, the os may easily be reached, and the hard round head of the child be felt without difficulty. Should a hard presenting part not be felt either through the dilated os or the walls of the uterus, it may be because there is a breech or body presentation, or there may be twins, or there may be an unusual amount of water in the uterus, or the child may have hydrocephalus—in either of these cases it might not be possible to decide immediately about the presentation and position.

FACE PRESENTATIONS cannot be detected very early in the labor. Before the membranes are ruptured the head is high and difficult of access. When it is reached the forehead is first encountered, afterwards we may feel the nose and mouth. It is unfortunate for us that we cannot usually distinguish a face presentation in the early stage of labor. It is not so important that we make an early diagnosis of presentation of the breech, as there is no danger to the mother involved in the latter.

PRESENTATION OF THE BODY should always be detected early, at least as soon as the membranes are ruptured. The abdomen of the mother is much longer in the transverse diameter than is usual, and the head of the child may sometimes be felt in the iliac fossa. The form of the mother's abdomen is irregular as the fœtus lies curved on itself. When we are able to touch the fœtus, if the shoulder presents, we first feel a small bony projection, the acromion point of the shoulder; then other points, including the acute angle of the shoulder blade. We should ascertain as soon as possible on which side the head lies, and also the posterior plane of the child.

Sometimes the hand comes down in the vagina or even appears at the vulva; if it does we may know by that (and by slipping the finger of our hand up into the axillary space) just how the child lies. If the back of the child's hand is turned towards the mother's right thigh the head is to the right, and if to the left thigh, to the left. The little finger being towards the coccyx indicates that the child's back is towards the mother's loins, and the same finger being towards the pubis is evidence that this is in front. It is quite important that these points should be noted.

There are various causes of tedious, difficult and obstructed labor, and in each case we are obliged to depend principally upon the touch for diagnosis. In some instances the difficulty will be obvious as soon as we attempt to make an examination. A NARROW and UNDILATABLE VAGINA will be easily recognized, but this will rarely be found a serious obstacle to the passage of the child; as the labor proceeds the vagina seems naturally to dilate and to be more softened and relaxed.

Cases have been reported where there was a *scirrhus tumor* or cancer connected with the neck of the uterus, even during labor; happily such cases are rare. The scirrhus would be felt hard and unyielding. A tumor of any kind connected with the os uteri, the vagina or the rectum may obstruct the descent of the child's head more or less according to its size and mobility. Of course they can be detected.

A VAGINAL CYSTOCELE ought always to be rectified. It sometimes happens that the bladder is caught by the head of the child in its descent into the cavity of the pelvis and pushed before it, and it can be seen as a soft red tumor between the vulva. The finger can be passed posterior to it, but not anterior, and the catheter cannot be passed in the usual direction.

A few cases are on record where a *stone* (calculus) in the bladder was pushed down before the fœtal head. A careful examination will show that the tumor is covered by the bladder; its hardness will indicate its nature.

A COLLECTION OF HARDENED FECES IN THE RECTUM is detected without difficulty. It will be of an irregular form, hard and inelastic.

SWELLING OF THE SOFT PARTS may cause obstruction. If the child's head is detained for a long time pressing upon the brim of the pelvis, it may obstruct the circulation and diminish the capacity of the passage. In such cases there is unusual heat and dryness in the parts.

When a nurse or midwife makes an examination by touching, she needs to continue it through several pains, and to repeat it again soon to know if there is any progress to the labor. If the progress is very slow this may be from various causes, some of which I will now simply name. It may be because the uterus is very much distended, and this renders the pains inefficient; there may be partial and irregular contractions of the uterus, weakness of constitution, fever or local inflammation, a want of irritability in the constitution, a deformity of the pelvis and spine, or doubts and fears on the part of the patient may diminish the action of the uterus. The labor may be slow because it is the first one, or because the membranes were ruptured too early, or because the woman is advanced in years at the time of having her first confinement. The uterus may be pitched over obliquely, there may be extreme rigidity of the os uteri, extreme rigidity of the soft parts of the mother, a contracted or small pelvis, the head of the child may be large and ossified so as to be unyielding. One or both arms may come down by the side of the head of the child; on the part of the mother there may be a distended bladder from inability to void the urine, there may be cicatrices (scars) or adhesions of the vagina, and in some cases it has happened that an enlarged ovary has dropped down into the pelvis, or a portion of intestine containing scybala or hardened feces obstructs the passage, or the os uteri is very minute, or imperforate, or totally absent.

Some of these cases may demand the interference of art in the first stage of labor, but delay at that time involves very little danger; as a rule neither the mother nor child is in danger (except when there is hemorrhage or convulsions) on account of labor before the membranes are broken. If the nurse can ascertain the cause of the delay and finds that time is what is especially needed, she must exercise patience herself and encourage her patient to do so.

It is hardly possible to predict beforehand in what cases convulsions will occur, but if there is much headache in the commencement of labor and if there has been considerable albumen in the urine of the patient, we have especial reason to apprehend trouble of that kind.

The history of the case is important in forming an opinion as to whether there may be severe hemorrhage. Some women are naturally predisposed to flowing.

CHAPTER I.
PRELIMINARY INSTRUCTION TO THE NURSE MIDWIFE.

It is my design in giving the following instructions to prepare the student of this work to be a skilled or skillful nurse, not to be simply a midwife; to act in conjunction with, not in opposition to, physicians; to conform to, and not to violate laws which regulate the practice of medicine; to officiate in cases of easy, natural labor sometimes, but never in cases requiring the use of instruments; to be prepared to act in emergencies until the doctor can come and take the case; not to treat the case when the services of a physician can be obtained and is desired or needed; in short to act intelligently in all cases in which women now act perhaps blindly, hurriedly and ignorantly.

The present state of feeling among our people, and especially among the medical profession in this country, would not sanction an effort to educate women solely as midwives.

But there is a general feeling or sentiment that every young lady ought to have that kind of education which may render her useful; that she should be prepared in some way to minister to the desires, wants and needs of her fellow creatures, and that some part of that knowledge or skill should be of that kind which would be available if these persons were thrown on their own resources; hence I would have some of you to be, not only nurses of the sick, but skilled nurses of lying-in women. And should some young lady after studying this work, decide to pursue the study of medicine thoroughly and become a physician, the knowledge here obtained would be available.

PRELIMINARY INSTRUCTIONS.

1. Do not stop short of a thorough knowledge of this book, every part of it.

2. Endeavor here to get a knowledge of midwifery that will qualify you to attend ordinary cases of *natural* labor, and enable you sometimes to give medicine when needed, and when there are no physicians in attendance; but understand that there are many times when the only proper thing for you to do is to send for a physician or experienced accoucheur.

3. Do not hesitate to seek knowledge and experience and instruction from any source where you think that you can obtain it. Physicians will be willing to aid you, and I think the time is coming when he will regard the educated nurse as his friend, and not as his natural enemy.

4. I do not think it best that you should call yourself a midwife, because if you do it will excite misapprehension and prejudice. Seek in every way to be skillful as a nurse, and seek to have a corresponding reputation.

5. Do not undervalue your position, if you have the wisdom and courage and perseverance necessary to prepare you to minister to your sex in their time of greatest suffering and trial. Do not doubt that your mission is an honorable one. And even if you do not minister very often to the sick in labor, except as the right arm of the medical man, you may help to raise the standard qualifications of the nurses of our land. Do not suppose that I am complaining harshly of our present supply of nurses. Women have shown a wonderful adaptability to the needs and exigencies of their suffering friends in nursing and caring for them. And it is because they are so ready to receive instruction that I endeavor here to furnish good instruction for them.

6. Do not suppose that your knowledge obtained by study is sufficient to enable you to act as midwife (except in an emergency), unless your studies are supplemented by observation, as mother nurse, &c.

7. Do not be unwilling to minister to women who are poor. The young physician is willing to do something in this way to gain experience and for the sake of humanity, and this will be your opportunity to gain experience without coming in competition with rivals.

8. The nurse as well as the medical man, must study the phenomena of labor at the bedside of the patient. No one can be qualified by mere reading for the duties of a midwife, and no woman that is diligent and observing can attend a case of labor without some addition to her knowledge.

INSTRUCTION TO THE NURSE MIDWIFE.

When I use the term nurse midwife I mean a nurse that has some knowledge of midwifery, that can be called to attend to women near the time that she expects to be confined, and that can remain in attendance for two weeks or more if it is desired or necessary. Sometimes a woman would, if possible, have a skilled nurse with her a week or more before confinement, especially because she would thereby avoid sending for the physician unnecessarily, and because she would be less likely to detain him for a long period of time.

If the nurse midwife understands her business she will in some cases do better for the woman than a physician in the commencement of labor. For instance, suppose that a doctor is called a distance of five miles and away from his home and his other patients, and when he examines the case the pains seem to be of the character of false labor pains. He knows that the real good of the patient might require that she should take an opiate, but the doctor would be unwilling to give it lest it might protract a real labor, and subject all parties to the inconveniences of a prolonged labor including unnecessary visits of the doctor. The nurse who can remain with the patient, if the labor should not be concluded in several days, would be more likely to do just what the good of the woman requires. And in such a case a skilled nurse would be peculiarly acceptable to a physician if he chanced to be called, because he would be much more at liberty to leave his patient if it seemed necessary to do so.

When a nurse midwife is called to attend a case, she should carry with her besides disinfectants, a male catheter, some laudanum or other opiate, quinine, and extract ergot, in order to be prepared for emergencies. Ordinary cases may require no medicine, but some cases do.

CHAPTER II.
THE NATURAL LABOR.

A NATURAL LABOR has been described as one "in which the head presents, and descends regularly into the pelvis; where the progress is uncomplicated, and concluded by the natural powers within twenty-four hours, (each stage being of due proportion), with safety to the mother and child, and in which the placenta is expelled in due time."

A skillful, careful examination in the commencement of labor will enable you perhaps to decide whether the labor will be natural or otherwise. But it may be your duty first to know if your patient is in ordinary health, or if she have any fever or organic disease, and you should enquire about the bodily functions generally, the condition of the pulse, skin, &c. Before making a digital examination you should notice the character of the pains, their frequency, force and regularity, the amount of voluntary effort, the character of the outcry, &c. From these enquiries you probably will be able to decide whether she is suffering from real labor, or false pains.

She will, however, probably not object to a digital examination and your opinion will be founded principally upon that. The modern practice is to wash the hands in antiseptic soap or some solution before making an examination.

We are directed by most writers to have the patient lie upon her left side near the edge of the bed when we examine her. The fore finger of the right hand (sometimes the left) after being well oiled or soaped should be passed along the perineum into the vaginal orifice, and is to be pressed upward and backward towards the promontory of the sacrum until the os uteri or the presenting part is found. Sometimes this is not reached without an effort. When reached endeavor to find the fœtal head or to determine what is the presenting part—feel sufficiently to distinguish the lips of the os uteri from the presenting portion of the fœtus. Do not be hasty in making the examination; wait till you examine sufficiently to know if the child is forced down; observe both during the time of a pain and during an interval, and observe if the pains dilate the os. Sometimes during a natural labor there may be a severe pain, and when the pain is hardest, the os contracts. By waiting to take a number of pains you will learn if there is real progress. When examining, note the calibre, heat and moisture of the vagina; the general condition of the cervix; the dilatability of the os uteri and the actual dilatation by the bag of waters or the fœtal head during a pain. If the head presents you can best learn the particular position when the pain is off; and after the membranes are ruptured you can decide better than previously. Ordinarily the sagittal suture can be felt, and perhaps both fontanelles, but you must not be discouraged at all if you cannot determine the exact position. Doctors ordinarily do not deem it necessary.

If you can decide that it is a head presentation and that the woman is undoubtedly in labor, you may probably decide that the labor will be natural, and you may properly tell the friends so, adding perhaps, that it will depend upon the character of the ensuing pains whether the labor will be protracted or short.

Various circumstances of which you are possibly not yet cognizant may make your case of labor a tedious or difficult one. You have decided, perhaps, that there is no obstruction to the passage of the child, no deformity of the pelvis, scirrhus or other tumors in the vagina, no cystocele, no prolapsed ovary, and that there is not a rigid perineum or imperforate vagina. If there is, you need to have a medical man present, but should none be obtained you will need to repeat your examination from time to time. Observe if each pain presses down the bag of waters and dilates the mouth of the womb, and if the soft parts are in a relaxed state, and if there is a show. Even if the appearances are thus promising, the labor may be slow and tedious from various causes.

1. Possibly hardened feces maybe in the rectum; if they are you may be assured of the fact when you make a digital examination, as they seem like tumors posterior to the vagina. The remedies are physic, enemas, rest—possibly opium.

2. Inefficient pains may be due to a bladder distended with urine. When this is suspected we should observe whether there is abdominal swelling (not tympanitic) low down; pain on pressure which gives rise to a desire to urinate; a constant desire to pass water though the patient has just performed the act, or a dribbling of water from the parts. If the bladder cannot otherwise be relieved a catheter should be used, and as a precaution to avoid wetting the bedclothes it is well to have a catheter made long enough by affixing a piece of India rubber tubing to the end of it to reach a vessel at the side of the bed. Never use force in passing a catheter in. It is very seldom that it is necessary to use it at all during labor.

3. If there is a hernial protrusion of the bowel, or a calculus of the bladder falling down in the passage you will probably have a medical man to officiate. But I may say that if there is need of your doing anything to replace them, or if it is necessary to return a prolapsed bladder, you can best do it when your patient is in the knee-chest position.

4. The lack of expulsive power is sometimes due to the want of sleep. If the first stage, that of dilatation, is prolonged the subsequent uterine contractions seem to want efficiency. In such cases if the patient can have a dose of opium or morphine administered to induce sleep it acts favorably. Where there is nervous excitement particularly, the efficiency of the pains are increased if we give opium and first procure a period of rest.

5. The uterus may be greatly distended and its expulsory power thereby weakened. In such cases there may be a suspension of the action of the uterus for several hours although the labor before that had made considerable progress. If pains of labor are feeble or slow or suspended, no harm can come to the mother or child (in such cases) except that the mother is compelled to bear them for a longer time. The only remedy that I would suggest is that the distention be relieved by the rupture of the membranes and discharge of water. If more efficient pains did not come on, then I would give a dose of morphine, which would either increase the pains, or give a period of rest.

6. Sometimes there are vehement and cramp-like pains in the abdomen producing no effect that is good and adequate, caused by partial irregular or spasmodic contractions of the uterus—usually what are called hour-glass contractions. If the bowels have been evacuated and there is no improvement, I would give one-fourth grain of morphine which will enable the woman to go through her labor more easily, and perhaps quite as quickly.

7. It is generally believed that a cord being very short and being around the neck of the child may protract a labor. I do not deny that this may possibly occur, and when the child's head is born, and I find that there is a coil of the funis on its neck I loosen it.

8. Weakness of the constitution when the general health of the woman is below the natural proper standard may be a cause why the uterine contractions are not severe. But in such cases the parts are not rigid, and nothing more than a dose of four or five grains of quinine is needed to make the pains effectual.

9. A want of irritability in the constitution frequently observed in fat and inactive women, or in those who are exceedingly timid, will sometimes be a cause of slow and lingering labor. Fear often lessens the energy of all the powers of the constitution, and diminishes or wholly suppresses for a time the action of all the parts concerned in parturition. Attendants should endeavor to inspire such patients with activity and resolution, and remove all fear from their minds. These cases are not dangerous but I have often found it necessary in this kind of cases to apply forceps. The skilled nurse might perhaps give eight or ten grains of quinine, if no physician has charge of the case.

10. Every woman is expected to suffer greater pain and to have a more tedious labor with her first child, and if a woman be advanced in age at the time of having her first child the difficulty attending her labor may be somewhat greater. A longer time may be required for the completion of the labor than in ordinary cases, but I do not advise giving any medicine unless it is perhaps a dose of quinine. There may be a little more need of assistance by instruments, &c.

11. An oblique position of the os uteri, it being projected on one side or the other of the center of the superior strait, or so far backwards that it cannot be felt for several hours after labor has begun, is a cause of delay. The presenting part may be found pressing against the walls of the pelvis at one point, instead of keeping its course in the center of the pelvic cavity. You should endeavor to place the patient so as to remedy this condition. When the presenting part is found to one side, it will be found that the fundus of the womb is lying to the opposite side; this should be remedied by a proper support of the abdominal tumor or by holding it up by the hands. For example, if the os uteri be projected to the left side, she ought to rest on the right side and have a pillow placed under her body; some physicians would prefer that she lay on the left side, but without the pillow under her.

12. Extreme rigidity of the os uteri is a cause of tedious and very painful labors. It sometimes happens that the os is dilatable, but the pains are not sufficiently expulsive. Perhaps at the same time the os is found far back towards the promontory of the sacrum, and the head appears not to be driven directly into the os so as to aid in its dilatation, but rather presses against the anterior wall of the cervix. In such a case the end of the finger can be hooked into the anterior lip of the os uteri so as to aid in the

dilatation, and also to help correct the displacement of the os. In other cases we may help dilate the os by a firm and gentle sweep of the finger around the advancing part of the child's head within the os. But we cannot always do this, because we may be afraid of rupturing the membranes prematurely. If the membranes have been already ruptured, we may act more boldly, but we must never make any great efforts to dilate it artificially lest we excite inflammation. In many cases it is best to give ¼ gr. of morphine, and inform the suffering woman that she cannot possibly get through her labor in a short time, but if you can give her an hours' rest, the os, which is rigid, will be more relaxed and pains more effectual.

13. In first labors there is sometimes unusual rigidity of the soft parts, which are external. Where the perineum is rigid it may require several hours continuance of the pains before it is sufficiently stretched to allow the head of the child to pass. But the difficulty can hardly be relieved by our interposition. We should generally wait the due time, as we must also if the os coccygis is anchylosed with the sacrum.

14. The head of the child may be comparatively large when the pelvis is of the ordinary form and size. This may be a cause of delay though it may perhaps cause nothing more than prolonged, tedious labor. In such cases you have time to send for a doctor, even if he lives at a distance. After the woman has been a long time in labor he will think it best to apply the forceps.

You will be importuned in cases of slow and tedious labor to administer ergot, but any one who knows the action of the drug would never give it in any of the following cases: 1. Where the os is not well dilated. 2. When any mechanical obstacle exists to the passage of the child, or when there is a tendency to convulsions, and *you* should never give ergot except for hemorrhage; and when you have much reason to fear it, you may in such cases give one or two twenty drop doses of the fluid extract very near the termination of labor. Quinine may be given as an oxytocic with safety. Morphine is liable to render the pains weak for a time, but it often increases their efficiency.

I will now enumerate your duties when you act as accoucheur.

1. Ascertain if the lady is really in labor. Make a digital examination. If the os is high up so as to be reached with difficulty, slightly patulous and rigid, and the pains are felt in front, there is reason to believe that the labor has not yet commenced—that she only has false labor pains. At this time

attend to the bowels; give perhaps paregoric or morphine to relieve her of what is to her useless and exhausting agony, and enjoin rest. You may at this time properly give her an enema containing ¼ of a grain of morphine or fifteen grains of chloral dissolved in gruel or starch or mucilage.

2. When you make an examination and find that the pains are efficient in producing a dilatation of the os uteri, that the parts are soft and relaxed, if there is a secretion called the show, if there is a favorable presentation, and the labor is making some progress, the patient should be told of all that is favorable in the case.

3. Be careful in making early examinations to, first, if possible, reach the os with the finger. When your finger presses against the cervix it will hurt her considerably more than it will when it presses against the presenting part of the child. 2. Avoid rupturing the membranes. 3. Notice if there is anything observable to hinder the progress of the labor. 4. Note any progress of the labor.

4. If everything is favorable, assure the patient of the fact; if you have doubts and fears upon some point, you need not express all your fear, but do not delay to send for a physician.

5. You may in the early stage of labor, permit the patient to move about as she wishes, and she may rest on the sofa when tired. She may have her usual diet, but not any stimulants.

6. From time to time make an examination. If the os is dilatable you need not fear that the membranes may then be ruptured. Learn as fully as possible the presentation and position, and if you press your finger against the child's head you may thereby reinforce weak pains.

7. Do not annoy the patient by pressing upon the back or anywhere during a pain if she requests you not to, but when she does not object you can make such pressure as will reinforce the action of the abdominal muscles. When she is lying on her back with her shoulders elevated so that she is in an almost vertical position, you can stand beside her with your back towards her head, and make the necessary palpation by pressing with your hands on her abdomen, one of them on each side. Do this only when there is no tenderness, when the os is dilated, when there is a normal pelvic canal and a low position of the presenting part. Seek in thus pressing to move the uterus to the axis of the pelvic brim, then with the palms of your hands to the sides or fundus of the uterus press gradually downward, increasing the pressure for six or eight seconds, and then gradually

diminishing. You may repeat this as often as she has a pain, and with an increasing force, and if the patient assents, you may make such pressure unremitting.

8. When the os uteri is fully dilated or soft and dilatable, the membranes may be broken by pressing with the end of your finger against it, or if this does not suffice, the finger nail previously nicked may open it.

9. When free hemorrhage occurs prior to delivery, it may depend upon placenta previa; that is, upon the placenta being attached very near or over the mouth of the womb; in such a case obtain a physician to take charge of the case if possible. You may yourself give half a teaspoonful of extract of ergot in the emergency.

10. During the progress of the labor you must always remember that the unassisted, natural powers are in most instances fully sufficient to bring the labor to a safe termination, and whatever you do should be of the kind that is not harmful. The important thing for the attendants to possess is gentleness and patience, and it is a good thing for the patient if she can be kept tranquil and cheerful.

11. A little light food may be offered the patient at any time during labor.

12. During the first stage of labor the patient must not strain or bear down to the pains, but it is my practice when I examine my patient and find that the head has not yet entered the pelvis, at the same time that the touch stimulates the uterus to contract, I direct the patient to bear down during each pain. After the head is fully engaged in the bones, no stimulus to pain is needed; however, as the bearing down pains come on, she should be advised to strain or press down.

13. Towards the last, when she is in great pain, if she be inclined to cry out, let her do so; never reprove her.

14. I approve of giving chloroform in some cases, but I do not advise the skilled nurse to give it except when a physician is present to direct its use.

15. During the latter part of the labor the only assistance you can render the woman is to support the back, and to give her something to pull upon if she is so inclined. A sheet tied to the foot of the bed may be useful for this purpose. At the very last, bearing down efforts should be discouraged.

16. When the head is about to be expelled we always fear there may be slight or severe lacerations of the perineum. Do not in any way hasten the expulsion, even if there should be a number of pains in which a part of the head presents externally during the pain, and then recedes when the pain goes off. I have not always been able to prevent laceration, but the following directions are the best that I can give: Endeavor to have the patient extend her legs, and do not have her knees drawn up close to the body at the last. When the perineum is put on the stretch, place the thumb and forefinger of the right hand on either side of the perineum, and press so as to aid the stretching or distention. When the perineum is distended and protruding you may cover the hand with a soft napkin and apply it across the perineum, also by the sides of the vulva, and make firm, moderate pressure during the pain. Endeavor to have the pressure equable around the head of the child.

17. When the head is expelled an attendant should make steady gentle pressure upon the uterus and follow it down, keeping her hand firmly upon it for several minutes, perhaps for half an hour, or if you have given a little attention to the child, you yourself may put your hand on the contracted uterus and firmly knead it for ten minutes.

18. It is not necessary to extract the body immediately after the expulsion of the head. It is better to wait three or four minutes for the return of a pain before making any traction.

19. Although a little traction can be made on the head, it is a better way while an attendant presses on the uterus, and while you hold on to the child's head with one hand, insert a finger of the other hand into the axilla, (under the child's arm) and gently extract the body.

20. The child may be born apparently asphyxiated—its face swollen—and of a dark livid color, and at first make only feeble and gasping efforts at respiration; if there is the least beating of the heart can be perceived, there is fair hopes of its recovery. The cord should at once be tied and the child removed from the mother. If one or two slaps on its body does not make it cry, try immediately artificial respiration by the Sylvester method perhaps, not omitting at first and afterwards to throw a little cold water on its body. If these efforts fail I would try to induce respiration by placing my hand over its nostrils and blowing into its mouth, and immediately afterwards compressing its lungs.

21. As soon as the child cries, as it most generally will as soon as it is born, proceed to tie and separate the cord. Tie the cord tight, so that it is thoroughly compressed and the vessels obliterated, applying the ligature about one and a half inches from the child, and then cut the cord one inch further from the child. The child can be rolled in flannel and removed, and you can attend to the mother and to the removal of the afterbirth.

22. In only a very few cases I have had post partem hemorrhage or adherent placenta to trouble me, and I commend to you the method that I have used for the removal of the placenta. I do not tie the cord until circulation has ceased in it. I then sever it, and usually two or three ounces of blood may flow from it. This I suffer to run into some vessel to avoid soiling the bed uselessly, and then wind the cord around my right hand so that I can hold it. If I cannot have an attendant to make proper pressure on the uterus, I immediately endeavor to compress it as much as I possibly can with my left hand, but I make very little traction on the cord. I usually instruct some one else to make strong and firm pressure upon the uterus, and I pass two fingers of one hand into the vagina, and learn thereby when the placenta descends, and if necessary assist in its removal. Although we should never hurry in removing the afterbirth, I believe that it always is easily removed if we make the effort very soon after the child is born, and if it is necessary for you to pass your hand into the uterus you can do so then better than at any other time. Judging from my own experience in cases of retained placenta, if you pass your hand along the cord into the uterus, you will find that an hour-glass contraction retains the afterbirth (whether adherent or not) in the fundus. You will have to press your fingers through the constricted portion and grasp it, and you can remove it steadily and slowly, but not stopping to give it "one or two turns in the vagina."

23. POST PARTEM HEMORRHAGE is liable to occur; when it does, obtain a physician as soon as you can, but some things must be done immediately. 1. Some one must grasp and compress the womb continually. 2. Remove the pillows and raise the foot of the bed so that the patient's body lies higher than her head. 3. If you have it, give a small teaspoonful of extract of ergot, or twenty drops spirits turpentine or (F. 96.) 4. Examine to know if possible, the source of the hemorrhage; if it comes from the vagina or perineum where there is laceration, it is not very dangerous. Inject hot water of the temperature of 115° into the uterus, and apply a dry cotton cloth, heated as hot as possible, to the abdomen externally. 5. Before using the injections

remove all clots from the vagina. 6. Quinine and stimulants may be exhibited if there is sinking, and ice may be applied to the abdomen and to the internal surface of the uterus, if the bleeding continues. I will here direct another thing which is very effectual, and which might be used at first in preference to anything else. 7. After removing the clots take a handkerchief or piece of muslin, saturated with vinegar, in your hand, pass it entirely into the uterus, and let it remain there 15 or 20 minutes, and your hand also. Your hand will compress the open blood vessels, and keep a clot in the mouth of them, and the vinegar will act as the best astringent that can be used. In one case of violent flooding I simply *held my hand still* in the uterus for five minutes, and the flow ceased. After the hemorrhage subsides you must be careful not to raise the patient's head above the level suddenly; her life may be put in jeopardy by suddenly raising her so that she sits up.

AFTER PAINS are very seldom severe in primapara cases, and they are less likely to be severe if the proper manipulations have compelled the womb to close completely, expelling all clots, &c. But sometimes there is a peculiar irritability or neuralgic condition of the womb which gives rise to excruciating pains. Ordinarily you may use Tully's powder. (F. 123, 93, 95, 107.)

RETENTION OF URINE in some cases necessitates repeated visits of the physician, and he will appreciate a nurse who can introduce the catheter. If the patient cannot at first void the urine, perhaps the application of a hot wet sponge over the pubis may enable her to do so. But it may be necessary to introduce a catheter two or three times a day until she regains her power over her bladder, or until the swelling of the urethra subsides.

It is well for the nurse to know that owing to the distensible state of the abdominal parietes, the patient will lay twelve or fourteen hours, perhaps, after the child is born, without manifesting a desire to void the urine, though her bladder may be very full, and you should remind her of the necessity of passing the water, lest it produce cystitis. In some instances the urethra and neck of the bladder are extremely irritable, causing strangury, and there may be some difficulty in passing the catheter, but the urine must be evacuated, and afterwards it may be necessary to use ergot, laxatives, opiates and fomentations. (F. 125, 126, 162.)

CHAPTER III.
CONVALESCENCE.

VARIATIONS FROM ORDINARY CONVALESCENCE will, under ordinary circumstances, receive necessary attention from the physician, but the skilled nurse should know as much about them as possible, and I here make a brief reference to some of them.

The NERVOUS SHOCK, caused by the last pains of labor, in some cases is very severe. This is indicated not only by the exhaustion, but by the countenance which is expressive of suffering, anxiety and oppression. The pulse may be very slow or unusually rapid, the breathing may be panting. Opium is the best remedy, and this may be given in small doses repeated, or a teaspoonful of paragoric may be given, also aromatic ammonia, and 3 or 4 drops of spirits of camphor.

The STATE OF THE PULSE after a natural labor soon comes down to near the ordinary standard; if it remains above a hundred it is because there is some special cause. It will be quick if there are very hard afterpains, a tendency to flooding, diarrhœa or disturbance of the stomach, and it is quickened also when lactation commences.

The LOCHIAL DISCHARGE ordinarily continues about three weeks, at first of pure blood mixed with coagula, and if good uterine contraction has not been secured, coagula may be expelled for several days after the delivery. Sometimes there is a SUDDEN DECREASE OF THE LOCHIA, perhaps on the fifth and sixth day, and at the same time an increased bulk of the womb, and increased frequency of the pulse. Apply hot fomentations to the abdomen, and probably some clots will be expelled, but at the same time give purgative enemata; and if there is abdominal tenderness give an aromatic purgative and laudanum. (F. 108, 122). There are remarkable differences in the QUANTITY, QUALITY AND ODOR OF THE LOCHIA without any morbid affection of the uterus or vagina. But when the lochia are acrid, the vagina, labia and external parts become excoriated, and smarting or itching is caused. Try extreme cleanliness, frequent bathing, lead lotions, black wash, vaginal injections of warm water, and F. 153, 154.

If the discharge ceases a few hours after birth, or if it continues the usual time, but in very small quantity, or if it is prolonged beyond the usual period, or if it is excessive at first, and if at the same time all the other symptoms are favorable, there is not occasion for much medicine, though it may be necessary to give the patient a better diet, possibly some tonics. (F. 174, 175). It sometimes occurs that the lochia is suddenly discharged in double quantity after the patient is permitted to sit up or walk about. In such cases enjoin extra rest.

If the red discharge continues longer than usual, or if it return after yellow or greenish discharges, you should be on your guard against HEMORRHAGE. Enjoin rest in a horizontal position under light clothing.

Occasionally the LOCHIA HAVE A VERY FETID ODOR. It is not very rare to observe a very disagreeable odor in the lochia without any bad results, but this often indicates the retention and putrefaction of coagula or a small portion of the placenta or membranes. Syringe out the vagina freely night and morning with Labaraques solution or some other antiseptic wash, (F. 153) and once or twice a day with warm milk and water. A weak solution of carbolic acid 1 in 50 may be used, and it may be proper to throw it into the uterus.

The SECRETION OF MILK generally becomes established in about forty-eight hours, and very often on the third day the breasts become turgid, hot and painful. There may, or may not, be some general disturbance, fever, chills, &c., but if there is it will usually be relieved after the milk is drawn out. It is customary on the morning of the third day to secure an action of the bowels, and this generally allays the vascular action if it is excessive. But very trivial causes may set up INFLAMMATION OF THE BREAST, and this is always liable to end in suppuration, which may be long continued and distressing.

The MAMMARY INFLAMMATION may follow exposure to cold, a blow or other injury on the breast, some temporary engorgement of the lacteal tubes, or sudden and depressing mental emotions, and it often follows from fissures and erosions of the nipples. To prevent the formation of an abscess, endeavor to remove the engorgement of the lacteal ducts by gentle hand friction with oil or F. 209, 202. Moderate the inflammation by giving five drops of the extract Phytolacca decandra (Poke root) every two hours—give saline cathartics, minute doses of aconite, and perhaps a large dose of quinine. Keep the patient in bed and have the affected breast supported by a suspensory bandage. Apply hot fomentations containing a solution of carbolic acid, or poultices containing it, and the breasts may be smeared with belladonna extract rubbed down with glycerine; or belladonna liniment or ointment may be applied (F. 201). Belladonna plasters or diachylon plasters may be useful. Give 15 grains bromide potassa.

WHEN PUS HAS FORMED notwithstanding efforts made to cure the inflammation, as soon as it is near the surface so that it can be detected by the fluctuation, the abscess should be opened. During the last few years careful surgeons have been unwilling to make any incision or lance even an ordinary abscess without employing some antiseptic method, such perhaps as the following:

The patient's skin where the incision is to be made, is first to be washed in 1 to 1000 bichloride of mercury solution—hands and instruments employed in the work must touch nothing that is not sterilized; hands must be washed in the same solution before operating—sponges that are used must be cleaned and stored in a 1 to 20 carbolic acid solution, and instruments must be soaked in the same for 15 minutes before being used, and some apply a large wad of bichloride of cotton or gauze to catch the exuded pus.

The following is Lister's antiseptic method which he first directed, to prevent the introduction of air containing living germs:

"A solution of one part of crystalized carbolic acid in four parts of boiled linseed oil having been prepared, a piece of rag from four to six inches square is dipped into the oily mixture and laid upon the skin where the incision is to be made. The lower edge of the rag being then raised a scalpel or bistoury dipped in the oil is plunged into the abscess and an opening about three-quarters of an inch in length is made, and the instant the knife is withdrawn the rag is dropped upon the skin as an antiseptic curtain, beneath which the pus flows out into a vessel placed to receive it, and all the pus should be pressed out as near as may be. For a dressing afterward Playfair recommends the following: About six teaspoonfuls of the above mentioned solution of carbolic acid in linseed oil is mixed up with common whiting to the consistence of firm paste; this is spread upon a piece of tin foil about six inches square, so as to form a layer about a quarter of an inch thick; the tin-foil thus spread with putty is placed upon the skin, so that the middle of it corresponds to the position of the incision, the antiseptic rag used in making the incision being removed the instant before. The tin-foil is then fixed securely by adhesive straps, the lower edge being left free for the escape of the discharge into a folded towel placed over it, and secured by a bandage. The dressing is changed once in twenty-four hours, as a general rule, and must be methodically done. A second similar piece of tin-foil having been spread with the putty, a piece of rag is dipped in the oily solution and placed on the incision the moment the first tin is removed. This prevents mischief during the cleaning of the skin with a dry cloth, and pressing out the discharge from the cavity."

The same author directs methodical strapping of the breast with adhesive plaster, in cases of long continued suppuration, and he adds that "much attention must be paid to general treatment, and abundance of nourishing food, appropriate stimulants and such medicine as iron and quinine will be indicated."

I give on the authority of another the following as good treatment for SORE NIPPLES:

"1. Keep everything that will irritate, whether clothing or medicine, away from the nipple, and have the excess of milk drawn from the breast in the easiest way possible. 2. Keep the excoriated nipple thickly covered with sub-nitrate of bismuth. 3. When the nipples are cracked at the base keep the cracks filled with bismuth, and put on a round piece of adhesive plaster starred in the centre, and just large enough to slip over the nipple and extend around its base an inch or more every way. When this is loosened it must be reapplied." (F. 231, 243).

There are certain accidents of parturition so grave in their nature, and attended by symptoms so alarming and urgent that no nurse would attempt to treat the patient except under the direction of a physician. I only refer to them because it is believed that some of these serious cases might have been prevented by early proper action on the part of the midwife or other attendant.

INVERSION OF THE UTERUS sometimes occurs, though but rarely. If it is in the practice of a midwife, and if she be at the time pulling on the cord, that will be assigned as the cause of the accident. Inversion consists essentially in the enlarged and empty uterus being either partially or entirely turned inside out. The immediate symptoms are those of shock or collapse— fainting, small, rapid and feeble pulse, possibly convulsions, or vomiting, and a cold, clammy skin. The countenance becomes deadly pale, the voice weak, and other symptoms indicates sudden exhaustion or sinking. In cases of partial inversion the symptoms are not so striking. Hemorrhage to a large amount, frequently but not always occurs. In more than half the cases no mechanical cause can be traced, but as it is sometimes attributed to pulling on the cord, to pressure with the hand on the fundus, and also to the patient straining forcibly, these combined causes should be avoided. When the symptoms named are present, you can give the patient some aromatic ammonia or other stimulant; always obtain a physician as soon as possible.

PUERPERAL MANIA is nearly always preceded by restlessness, want of sleep, and other premonitory symptoms. When the mania first comes on there is usually causeless dislike to those around her, and as the child may be the object of suspicion, the nurse must be extremely careful that the patient does not have an opportunity to seriously injure it. The course of treatment must be mainly directed to the maintenance of the strength of the patient, and the two things most needful are a sufficient quantity of suitable food and sleep. Possibly your efforts in this direction before the disease is fully developed, may ward off the disease.

PUERPERAL SEPTICEMIA was formerly called puerperal fever; as its nature is now better understood than formerly, we hope to do more than was formerly done to prevent it. This fever is now very generally believed to be produced by the absorption of septic matter into the system, through some tear or laceration in the generative tract such as exists after labor.

This septic matter may be from within the patient such as coagula, or membrane, or placenta partly decomposed; or from without as might be on the hands of physician and nurse, or in the air from cases of erysipelas, &c., or in some way from puerperal patients.

The notion that puerperal fever and septicemia is produced by BACTERIA has now become an established doctrine, and has given rise to a rational treatment based thereon, especially for their prevention.

As prophylactic means may be mentioned, the use of a carbolic solution 1 in 30 which the practitioner or nurse applies before touching any case, the use of carbolized oil 1 in 8 for lubricating the fingers, catheter, forceps, &c.; syringing out the vagina with diluted Condy's fluid, rigid attention to cleanliness in napkins, &c. The nurse should use antiseptics to only a very limited extent without the advice of a physician.

CHAPTER IV.
CARE OF INFANT CHILDREN.

Infants sometimes require treatment for ailments either slight or severe when the advice of a physician cannot be obtained.

The NAVAL is sometimes a little sore after the naval string comes away. It may be dressed by putting a little simple cerate or vaseline or carbolized cosmoline on lint or a linen rag, and applying it to the part affected every morning, and a bread poultice every night until it is quite healed.

A RUPTURE OF THE NAVAL is sometimes caused by much crying, and it may be occasioned by the nurse pulling on the cord to remove it before it will readily separate from the infant's body.

The best treatment is a piece of adhesive plaster as large as the top of a tumbler, with a properly adjusted pad made of several folds of muslin fastened on the plaster, which will keep the bowels from protruding. The bandage or belly band can be put on over this.

If the infant have a GROIN RUPTURE the only proper treatment is to keep on it day and night if it cry much, a well fitting truss. In applying the truss be careful to return the rupture thoroughly, and endeavor to have it well adjusted or it will chafe and will not effectually cure.

If the child is TONGUE TIED so that it cannot apply its tongue to the nipple to suck, the frenum may be cut, but it will not be necessary to make more than a small nick or a slight cut in it.

MILK IN THE BREASTS OF NEW BORN INFANTS, or a serous fluid resembling it, is often found, and sometimes there is considerable swelling both of the breasts of male and female children. It is not the better way to apply plasters or to squeeze or press them, but the milk may be drawn out by putting an open top thimble over the nipple and drawing on it.

CHAFINGS may be caused by inattention to cleanliness. Fat babies are subject to them, and when there is disorder of the bowels or kidneys they cannot at all times be prevented. Thoroughly sponge the parts with tepid rain water, allowing the water from a well filled sponge to stream over them, then carefully dry with a soft towel, and perhaps dust over them sub-nitrate of bismuth. (F. 202.)

DIARRHŒA and DYSENTERY and also COSTIVENESS are among the ailments with which infants may be afflicted. I wish to be particular in giving directions, that these may generally be avoided, but I must again repeat that the nurse should never be influenced by my advice to do any thing contrary to the directions of the attending physician.

To avoid the subsequent necessity of giving medicine you must be very careful in their administration at first. It is indeed necessary that the meconium should be purged off at first, but nature in general provides such physic as is required, and if the child is applied to the mother's breast, it obtains in the colostrum such medicine as it needs. Where the infant cannot obtain anything from the breast a gentle aperient may be given, and I name the following as being suitable: either molasses and water, raw sugar, a solution of manna in warm water, a teaspoonful of sweet oil, or of simple syrup of rhubarb, or in more obstinate cases, of castor oil, or one-fourth teaspoonful compound licorice powder, (F. 108.) but you must never give a drastic purgative, and you must not repeat the aperient if the discharges become yellow and natural. A young infant ought to have from three to six motions in the twenty-four hours, the color ought to be of a bright yellow or orange, and of the consistency of mustard as ordinarily prepared for the table, and there ought not to be any lumps or curds in its motions. A mother or nurse ought to be very observant of the state of the bladder and bowels—should inspect motions daily and see that they are not slimy, or curdled, or green. If they are she should be very careful, especially in regard to what the mother eats and drinks. If the bowels are costive she must avoid the frequent repetition of opening medicine, however gentle and well selected the aperients may be. They interfere with digestion, often irritate the bowels, and render them more costive. For the sake of the child as well as herself, the mother may vary her diet considerably after the first week, she may eat boiled and stewed, broiled and roast meats, mutton, lamb, and beef, fish, game, and chickens, potatoes, turnips, spinach, celery, peas, beans, figs, bananas, prunes, baked apples, &c. (F. 45 to 60.) The bowels of the child that nurses generally (not always) keep pace with those of the mother, and she must endeavor both for her own sake and that of the child, to keep her bowels loose by means of diet. If necessary she must take physic. (F. 107, 108, 109.)

If the constipated child nurses the mother and the mother constantly pays proper attention to her own health, and especially to her diet, the child will very seldom require physic. Indeed I would not give active physic when the child seemed well, if it did not have a passage oftener than once a week. If it has cow's milk or other food besides the mother's milk, do not boil the milk and you can add to the cow's milk, corn starch, or the following: Make a thin mush by boiling a small quantity at a time of unbolted wheat flour in water and straining it through a sieve while hot. The child may sometimes be fed with this alone, a little sweetened. Molasses may be given freely, or molasses and soda. The child should be watched, and if there is occasional costiveness, and at the time any indisposition, make a suppository of common soap about an inch in length and a quarter of an inch thick, dip it in water and pass it into the rectum. Or give an injection of less than a gill of water with perhaps a teaspoonful of molasses and a pinch of salt. But I would avoid the practice of giving an enema daily, as tending to get up a bad habit in the system. Should the costiveness have provoked fever, induced pain, or excited convulsions, active physic may be given, either castor oil, magnesia, calomel, or F. 108. But be sure that costiveness is not brought on by giving paregoric or other opiates, and let a child drink freely of pure cold and fresh water. The water may be boiled to destroy germs, and then cooled in a refrigerator; it should always be boiled before being used when there is an epidemic of bowel complaint prevailing.

In DYSENTERY there is a specific inflammation and ulceration of the mucous membrane of the colon, especially of the lower part, and of the rectum—there is generally some fever, frequent and bloody stools, tenesmus, and griping pains. Sometimes it attacks an infant or a delicate child, there being at first for several days diarrhœa, the motions being slimy and frothy like frogspawn, afterward entirely mucous and blood. The child is dreadfully griped, strains violently, and screams, and twists about every time it has a motion, and there is vomiting and great prostration.

You should in treating the child at the breast still keep him to it, and give it no other food. If the mother's milk is not good, procure if possible a healthy wet nurse. If the child must be fed give it cow's milk from one healthy cow—fresh from the cow—small quantities at a time and frequently, mixed with gum arabic water. In the commencement a warm bath may be used, or as a substitute you may wrap the child in a blanket that has been previously wrung out of hot water; over this put a dry blanket and keep the child thus enveloped for twenty or thirty minutes.

Formula 74 and 99 may be used, but the dose for a young child must be small to accord with its age.

CHOLERA INFANTUM is more prevalent in the United States than in any other country. The continued heat of summer is a predisposing cause, and improprieties in diet and clothing, worms, premature weaning, and teething are exciting causes.

You may treat this disease in the initial stage by giving F. 80, and also for a child a year old, injections of a gill of warm water in which a teaspoonful of common salt has been dissolved, allowing the patient three or four times a draught of warm water, as much as it desires to drink. Perhaps the drink will be immediately vomited, but it will at least remove irritating matter from the stomach. The injection, too, may operate immediately, but it may bring with it a fecal or bilious discharge, and if several times repeated, its effects will be salutary. A muslin cloth heated almost to scorching and applied once or twice dry to the neck, may stop vomiting, and draughts applied to the extremities may also be of much benefit. After using injections of warm soft water, anodyne injections may be given three or four times a day; but cases of this kind are too serious for any nurse or mother to treat, if the services of a physician can be obtained; and I will only mention one or two things more. When the extremities are cold put the child for a few minutes in a warm bath of mustard water, and then employ friction to the skin.

I have found chicken tea made by boiling the chicken very soon after it is killed, very useful in checking the vomiting and curing the child.

Of course a physician will be obtained in these serious cases if possible.

RETENTION OF URINE in the newly born infant if slight is easily removed by giving two or three drops of spirits of nitre once an hour in a little sweetened water, or if obstinate it may be aided by castor oil and the warm bath. A little pumpkin seed or parsley root tea also succeeds remarkably well.

APTHÆ is usually called the baby's sore mouth. It generally begins on the inner part of the lower lip or corner of the mouth, as a small white speck which resembles a coagulum of milk. These aphthous white pustules soon appear over the inside of the cheeks and on the tongue and gums. The eruption is very white and looks as if whey or curds were spread over the mouth, which is hot and painful, and the disease sometimes does, and at other times does not cause fever. I regard this complaint as being one of the germ diseases, although the fact has not yet been demonstrated. The children fed upon farinaceous food are most liable to this disease, and during its continuance, if the child is not at the breast it should be kept entirely to the milk of one cow. Medicine should be given with regard to the stomach and bowels. If the passages from the bowels are green, magnesia is a proper kind of physic, and when there is diarrhœa use formula 80, 77, 81.

GENUINE JAUNDICE may attack a young child, but this is to be distinguished from those cases where there is only a generally diffused YELLOW COLOR OF THE SKIN. In the latter class of cases there are no symptoms indicating any serious disease; the yellowness may continue for several days, and this disappears without the aid of any medicine and without leaving any evil behind. But in jaundice the whites of the eyes and the tears are tinged yellow, and, besides, the feces are paler than they should be, the urine is yellow, and other serious symptoms are added. If the bowels be costive, or irritated to frequent efforts, if the abdomen swells and becomes tense, if the child is uneasy and inclined to vomit, if it refuse the breast and frequently moans as if in pain, if it emaciate rapidly, jaundice in a bad form is present, and there is probable disease of the liver. Call the doctor.

I need not continue my instructions any farther in regard to the diseases of infancy, as you are expected to act as far as you can under the directions of a physician. But I must again advise you as to how you are to treat your medical advisor. Give him your entire confidence. Be truthful and candid with him. Have no reservations; give him a plain statement of the symptoms. Be prepared to state the exact time the child showed any illness. Tell him if the child had a chill; if there be any eruption on the skin, note the quantity and appearance of the urine, the number, color, &c., of the stools— all the symptoms of the disease. Strictly obey the doctor's orders in diet, in medicine, in everything, and never omit any of his suggestions. If the case be severe, never call a second physician without first consulting and advising with the one first chosen; speak in the presence of children with respect and reverence of the doctor, and endeavor to have them like him. Send for the doctor when practicable early in the morning, as the daylight is most favorable for making the examination, but if the illness come in the night do not delay on that account; if you do not know what to do, it is better that the doctor be called early than late.

CHAPTER V.
CASES OF DIFFICULT LABOR.

I wish to give you so much instruction in regard to cases of difficult labor that you may at least be prepared to decide in any case when the services of a physician is indispensably necessary, to decide whether the parturition in a given case is a natural one that does not need any assistance, or an unnatural one requiring the assistance of the art of midwifery, scientific or manual, for the relief of irregularities and difficulties. In general I shall adopt Churchill's divisions and definitions as I think they are very concise and correct.

TEDIOUSLABOR.

"DEFINITION. The head of the child presents and the labor is terminated without manual or instrumental assistance, but it is prolonged beyond twenty-four hours from causes which occasion delay in the first stage."

Prolongation of labor is of comparatively small consequence when the membranes are still intact, as they serve to protect the soft parts of the mother as well as the body of the child from injurious pressure, but the mere lengthening of the labor may become a serious thing when the head has entered the pelvis, when the uterus is strongly excited by reflex stimulation, and when the maternal soft parts as well as the fœtus and cord are exposed to severe pressure. When we find no evil resulting from the delay we need not interfere, but when we can remove the cause of it we are bound to do so.

In tedious labors the woman becomes fatigued, the loss of sleep is much felt, her spirits become depressed, and the stomach is more or less disturbed, but when the other bodily functions are performed regularly, the skin is cool, the pulse quiet, the tongue clean and moist, there is no headache, and the pains recur tolerably regularly, the condition of the patient is favorable, though the pains are inefficient and vary in their duration and frequency. There is usually loud outcry during the pain in the first stage of labor, but there is often sufficient remission of the suffering for the woman to get some quiet sleep, and generally there is progress to the labor.

INEFFICIENT ACTION OF THE UTERUS occurs most commonly in women confined for the first time, and sometimes we can ascribe it to no cause but constitutional peculiarity, or a deranged state of the digestive organs, or mental depression; in other cases it may be caused by irritation of the os and cervex uteri.

The skilled nurse may properly send for a medical man, though he is not indispensably necessary in such cases. The best thing which she can give in such cases is a quarter grain dose of morphine to suspend the pains and induce sleep, or if this is not thought best it may be proper to give physic or stimulating enemata. Never give ergot to increase the pains, but it may be proper to give several grains of quinine. However, giving medicine must be left as much as possible to the physician.

Excessive amount of liquor amnii with undue distention of the uterus in some cases renders the pains inefficient. The unusually large size, and the fluctuation of the abdominal tumor may be obvious, but although an accoucheur might deem it advisable to evacuate the waters, the skilled nurse who could not be certain that there was a favorable presentation, should not do it. She must exercise patience herself and encourage the patient to do so, and time will probably do the work, though it is better to commit the case to a doctor.

An undilatable os uteri, which remains rigid although the pains are severe, may sometimes be felt with its edges thin and stretched over the head, and sometimes thick and tough. In the majority of cases patience and time may overcome the obstacle, but as it is best in some cases to give chloroform, chloral, &c., and in some instances to use local means to relax or dilate the os, the physician should be sent for. The nurse may properly give the patient a hip bath.

Premature escape of the liquor amnii and obliquity of the uterus are both causes of tedious labor, but not cause for apprehension or special interference. I have already given some hints in regard to the treatment of the latter class of cases.

The posterior lip of the cervix uteri in some instances is retracted while the anterior is drawn tightly over the crown of the head. In such cases it has been my practice to draw with my finger the anterior lip forward, and during the time of the pain to press my finger against the head of the child. I do this believing that the anterior lip is caught between the head and symphasis pubis, and that it will be better retracted while support is given to the head.

POWERLESSLABOR.

"Definition. The labor is prolonged in the second stage by causes which act on the uterine powers primarily or secondarily, rendering the pains feeble and inefficient or totally suppressing them." In consequence of the stage at which the delay takes place, certain symptoms arise which render speedy delivery imperative.

The second stage may continue twenty hours or more without any bad symptoms, but usually if it exceeds twelve hours some of the following symptoms may be observed: The pains become irregular as to recurrence and force—perhaps become weaker—there may be rigors or shiverings—the vomiting may be distressing—there may be constant restlessness and fever—the vagina and uterus may be hot and tender to the touch—and the pressure of the child's head may prevent the evacuation of the bladder. The same causes (weak constitution, mental emotion, disease, &c.), which in the first stage rendered the labor tedious without bad symptoms, now occasion these and perhaps even more alarming indications. If an experienced accoucheur now arrives to take charge of the case he will be likely to apply the forceps, but it would have been better if he had been there and applied them sooner, before the patient had undergone so much suffering; and the midwife who attends a woman in the first stage of the labor should ascertain if any of the following causes of powerless labor exists: Is there a weak constitution or one exhausted by disease? Is it a first labor and the woman of advanced age? Has the patient had very many children? Is there excess of liquor amnii? Is there malposition of the uterus? No midwife should undertake to manage such a case alone.

OBSTRUCTEDLABOR.

"DEFINITION. The progress of the labor is impeded by some mechanical obstruction in the passages connected with the soft parts, which by causing delay in the second stage leads to the developement of symptoms of powerless labor."

The symptoms that arise and that cause anxiety are the same as in a case of powerless labor, except that while in the latter kind the pains are feeble, in the case of obstructed labor the pains may be vigorous and severe but ineffective in consequence of obstacles. I may say, however, that these obstacles have not been often met with in my practice. Since I commenced the practice of midwifery three thousand cases of pregnancy have been under my observation for treatment, and I have not yet met with any of the following causes of obstructed labor: Occlusion of the os uteri, cancer of the os uteri, undilatable vagina, tumors in the pelvis, or diseased ovary, stone in the bladder, imperforate hymen, hernial protrusion into the vagina, or blood effusions, or swelling of the soft parts. I have met with one case of excessive œdematous effusion of the vulva, which I relieved by puncturing the skin; one case of cystocele which I relieved by first drawing the water and then returning the bladder, before the head of the child descended into the pelvis; one case of ovarian tumor that was not at that time in the pelvis; one case of small fibrous tumor on the neck of the uterus, which did not much obstruct the labor; and numerous cases where hardened feces in the rectum was an obstacle until they were removed by the use of enemata. In cases of obstructed labor the skilled nurse will show her wisdom by detecting the obstructions and sending for an accoucheur.

DEFORMEDPEL VIS.

"DEFINITION. The progress of the labor impeded by abnormal deviations in the form of the pelvis, giving rise to delay in the second stage, or rendering the descent of the child impossible without assistance, or altogether impracticable. The symptoms are those of powerless labor."

The EQUALLY ENLARGED PELVIS, enlarged in all its parts, is not often met with, and is of no obstetric importance. If in any case this condition is diagnosed preceding or during labor, the patient should be watched by the nurse lest labor close so precipitately that the child falls to the ground.

THE EQUALLY CONTRACTED PELVIS—equally contracted in all its diameters, generally renders the labor difficult and tedious but not impracticable, by the natural powers. Other distortions such as has often been caused by rickets, &c., offer great obstruction to the passage of the child. In some cases a modification of the position of the child allows it to descend, but in many cases it is necessary to interfere and terminate the labor artificially. The nurse should not wait for unfavorable symptoms to appear before she sends for a man that is able to use the forceps, &c.

MALPOSITIONANDMALPRESENT ATIONOFTHE CHILD.

Unnatural or abnormal labor may be caused by some peculiarity on the part of the child, in the position or presentation. These cases demand the services of the skilled accoucheur, and I do not intend to hint that the nurse should ever attempt to do what an educated physician should be called to do in these cases.

FACE PRESENTATIONS sometimes retard the labor so much in the second stage as to give rise to unfavorable symptoms. In cases where the action of the uterus is so energetic as to finally expel the child, the sufferings of the mother are severe and prolonged. I have in my practice met with four cases, three of which were delivered by the natural powers, the children living; in one case craniotomy was performed. The mothers all lived. The diagnoses of face presentations is not easy at an early stage of labor. The finger first touches the forehead, which may be mistaken for the vertex. When the membranes are ruptured we may be able to make out the presentation. We may distinguish the edges of the orbits, the prominence of the nose, the mouth, &c. The bridge of the nose is the best guide, it being prominent, firm, and unlike any part of the breech or vertex. The face becomes tumefied during the labor, and the cheeks pressed together to resemble the nates, and it may be mistaken for a breech presentation. But in either presentation the proper course for the nurse is to leave the case alone in the expectation that the natural efforts will be sufficient to complete delivery. The child when born has a frightful appearance from the swelling and discoloration of one cheek, &c., but the injuries pass away in a day or two.

THE FOREHEAD TOWARDS THE ARCH OF THE PELVIS at the time of delivery is not favorable, but unless the pelvis is proportionately small no interference is necessary.

The BREECH may present at the brim in different positions, and the breech is distinguished by its roundness and softness, by the cleft between the buttocks, by the arms and by the organs of generation. In some cases the labor is concluded as quickly as if the head descended, in others it is more tedious. The results as regards the mother are as favorable as in head presentations. The danger to the child is in direct proportion to the length of time between the birth of the body and that of the head.

When the body is expelled so far as the umbilicus, the danger to the child commences, for at this time the cord may be pressed between the body of the child and the pelvic walls. A loop of the cord should be pulled down, and if it freely pulsates the child can probably be delivered alive.

Generally a judicious traction on the part of the accoucheur, combined with firm pressure through the abdomen applied by an assistant, will effect delivery of the head before the delay has had time to prove injurious to the child. If the arms of the child are above at the side of the head, the doctor will bring one down by passing a finger over the shoulder as near as possible to the elbow, and then drawing it across the face and chest until it arrives at the external orifice, but all this time it is the part of the nurse to continue to make effective pressure upon the abdomen of the mother—also while he delivers the shoulders—and while he perhaps introduces two fingers into the vagina of the mother to reach the upper jaw of the child and make pressure upon it, so as to depress the chin and facilitate the expulsion of the head.

PRESENTATION OF THE KNEES and PRESENTATION OF THE FEET is identical in its progress with breech cases, and the treatment of breech cases applies to footling presentations, but it is best to avoid pulling on the foot or feet that come down, as it is safer for the child if the lower part of the body is delivered quite slowly. Even if the nurse should in an emergency deliver the child, she should help principally by pressure on the mother's abdomen.

The only rule that I would have the skilled nurse adopt in regard to these cases, is that it is necessary that she should discover as early as possible if the labor is not a natural one, and if it is unnatural, should obtain the services of a physician as soon as possible. The same rule applies to cases of placenta previa hemorrhage, but I shall have more to say of these hereafter. A case of compound presentation where the hand and arm presents with the head, or in which the feet and hands, or one of each present together, also imperatively demand the services of an experienced accoucheur without delay. The nurse will be impotent to give any efficient help until the doctor arrives.

Presentation of the SUPERIOR EXTREMITIES will receive from me a full and complete description, because I believe that under certain circumstances the nurse should be prepared to operate by turning. As this radical opinion may perhaps be opposed by my medical brethren, I offer the following reasons for it which I consider a sufficient justification.

1. Cases of this class commence with the ordinary symptoms of labor; their peculiar character cannot usually be distinguished until the os is well dilated, and this is the only favorable time to perform the operation of turning.

2. Although in cities and villages generally, a physician's services can in most instances be immediately obtained, in the country it is not always practicable to obtain them within an hour or two of time.

3. Such knowledge as is necessary for the performance of this operation may be obtained from such description and instruction as can be given in books.

4. There are some women who possess the necessary traits of character, the complete exercise of their faculties, with the perfect coolness which is demanded of the operator in such a case.

5. I do not advocate trusting the operation to a nurse when the services of an accoucheur can possibly be obtained within the proper time.

6. The services of a physician, if obtained one or two hours after the arm is first thrust down in the vagina, may not be of any use because the time for turning is passed.

7. The operation of turning, performed by a properly instructed nurse, does not involve the least danger to the mother or child.

8. The only danger connected with this operation arises from the size of the hand of the operator, and the woman's hand is small.

9. It is a historical fact that at one period practitioners overrated the performance of turning, and extended its use to unsuitable cases, and after the invention of the forceps, they fell into an opposite error. It is possible that we may be in error if we hold that the nurse cannot be instructed to perform the operation of turning.

10. I do not advise that the nurse should ever attempt to turn in those cases in which the membranes have been long ruptured—the shoulder and arm pressed down into the pelvis, and the uterus contracted around the body of the child. I once succeeded in a case that two experienced physicians had tried in vain for several hours to turn, and I never had very much difficulty in turning, but there have been many cases where excellent operators could not succeed in turning.

In cases of PRESENTATION OF SHOULDER, ARM OR TRUNK, delivery by the natural powers is quite exceptional, though the natural powers have occasionally succeeded in expelling the child. The safety of the mother and child depend upon the early detection of the abnormal position of the fœtus, and upon their receiving proper treatment before labor has been long in progress.

The position of the child is one intermediate between the long and transverse diameters. It may lie with its back towards the abdomen of the mother or with the back towards the spine of the mother, and the head of the child may be towards the right or the left of the mother.

The existence of a shoulder presentation is not commonly suspected until the first examination is made during labor. Suspicion will arise from finding on examination that we are not able to reach the presenting part, and that the os uteri does not dilate as usual, and that when it becomes dilated the bag of membranes protrude of a conical form, but this is common to all malpresentations. When the shoulder has descended a little it is recognized as a round, smooth prominence, rounder than the elbow, and we may be able to reach the axilla, &c. The elbow may be recognized by the sharp prominence of the bone, and the hand can be distinguished from the foot by the fingers being wider apart and more readily separated from each other than the toes, and by the thumb which can be carried across the palm. The situation of the thumb and the aspect of the palm of the hand will mark whether it is the right hand or the left.

As soon as the nurse ascertains or suspects from an external palpation or a vaginal examination, that it is a cross birth she should send for the doctor, who ought to be there as soon as the membranes are ruptured, and the nurse must not be very persistent in making examinations lest she rupture the membranes prematurely. She may perhaps give a small dose of morphine, but I would not advise that she give chloroform as it is not necessary.

The right time to turn the child is when the os uteri is dilated, either before or immediately after the rupture of the membranes, and if a doctor cannot be soon obtained, it is better that a skilled nurse should turn the child, and if she is properly instructed, she should do it carefully and slowly, but without any fear and confidently. She can assure the patient that she will be able in a short time to relieve her sufferings.

In England the ordinary position for turning is on the left side. I prefer that the patient be placed across the bed on her back with her legs drawn up and supported by assistants. I now describe my own mode of operating.

I bare my right arm and hand (sometimes the left), lubricating it freely. If the waters have only recently escaped, and the os be dilated, the operation is performed with ease, especially after we have determined the position of the child.

I press the fingers together in the form of a cone, the thumb between the fingers—slowly and carefully press them into the vagina in an interval between the pains, and constantly and slowly press the hand in, only when the contractions of the uterus remit; never using any force, gently pass the fingers into the os; gently open the fingers a little occasionally to dilate the os sufficiently, and when it is expanded pass the hand into the uterus, make out the presentation accurately, so as to keep my hand to the abdomen of the child; always keep the hand still during a pain; when there is an interval between the pains, carefully search for the feet; when one of the feet is found, clasp the leg at the knee with one finger; flex the leg at the knee so that the finger has a good hold of it, draw it down in the absence of a pain; as the knee approaches the os when it is drawn down over the abdomen of the child, the shoulders and head recede towards the fundus, and when the head has reached the fundus and the knee is brought through the os, the case is converted into a knee presentation, and I deliver slowly but without needless delay—making a little traction during each pain, the management being conducted as in feet presentations, and the whole process being assisted by pressure made on the uterus by my left hand, or by the hand of an assistant.

Possibly these directions will be better understood if I use the language of another who directs:

1. That the patient be placed on her left side near the edge of the bed.

2. The os externum is then to be dilated with the fingers reduced into a conical form, acting with a semi rotary motion of the hand.

3. When the hand is passed through the os externum it must be slowly conducted to the os uteri. We may perforate the membranes with the finger if they are not broken.

4. The hand must then be passed along the thighs and legs of the child until we come to the feet. If both the feet lie together we must grasp them firmly with one hand, but if they are distant from each other we may deliver by one foot.

5. Before we begin to extract we must be sure that we do not mistake a hand for a foot. The feet must be brought down with a slow, waving motion into the pelvis, when we are to wait till the uterus contracts, still retaining them in the hand.

6. The feet are to be brought down with each return of the pain, and the labor may be finished partly by the efforts of the mother and partly by art.

7. If the toes are turned towards the pubis the back of the child is towards the back of the mother which is an unfavorable position.

8. If the toes are towards the sacrum, the back of the child is towards the abdomen of the mother, and this position is advantageous when the head comes to be extracted.

9. When the feet of the child has passed through the os externum, wrap them in a cloth and holding them firm wait till there is a pain, during the continuance of which gently draw down the feet. When the pain ceases we must rest, we merely assisting the efforts of the patient.

10. When the child is brought so low that the funis reaches the os externum, a small portion of it is to be brought out to slacken it, and from this time the operation is to be finished as speedily as it can be with safety, but if the circulation of the funis be undisturbed, there is no occasion for haste as the child is in safety.

11. If the child should stick at the shoulders the arms must be successively brought down.

12. When both the arms are brought down the body of the child must be supported upon our left arm and hand, the fingers on each side of the neck, and if the head should not come easily away, we must introduce the forefinger of one hand into the mouth of the child to render the position of the head more convenient for passing.

12. When a child has been extracted by the feet, the placenta usually separates very easily, but in the management we are to be guided by the general rules.

13. In these cases the child usually needs to be resuscitated, and the nurse should arrange so that hot and cold water may be at hand if required.

In these descriptions of the operation I have mentioned both the back and side as good positions for the mother, because some accoucheurs prefer one position and some the other. Some prefer to have the patient on the hands and knees. But if the nurse have the instructions here given well in her mind, she can operate in either position. If she ascertains at first how the child lies she may sometime reach its abdomen better if she introduces her left hand, but the main point is to proceed slowly and carefully. She should be careful in passing in her hand to change the direction of it in accordance with the pelvic axis, and should not use much force at any time. The danger to the mother is very small indeed; the danger to the child arises, as in breech presentations, from the compression of the funis, which commences about the time the buttocks appear at the os externum. But the safety is only when the operation is performed at the proper time. The nurse must never operate if the services of a physician can be obtained at that time, but when it is necessary she may proceed to turn, doing it slowly and properly, but fearlessly and confidently. If the doctor that is sent for is informed before he arrives that it is a case of hand presentation, he will come dreading the difficulties that he may encounter, and if he can have the satisfaction of knowing when he comes that the woman is safely delivered, he will be exceedingly glad.

CHAPTER VI.
CONCLUDING INSTRUCTIONS IN MIDWIFERY.

What I shall say of PLURAL BIRTHS, and MONSTERS, of CHILDREN AFFECTED WITH HYDROCEPHALUS, OR ASCITES, of EXCESSIVE SIZE OF THE FŒTUS, of DEFECTS IN THE FORMATION OF THE FŒTUS, of PROLAPSE OF THE FUNIS, &c., will be compressed in a few words. I am not instructing the nurse to attempt to conduct a case of even natural labor without having a physician if he can be obtained, but she should consider the services of a trained practitioner *imperatively* necessary in these unusual cases. In either instance there may be a safe delivery by the natural powers alone, and the nurse may act in an emergency, but it would not be consistent with the plan of this work for me to describe in detail the various operations that are sometimes performed in these several cases, or to give instructions in the use of instruments, which I advise the nurse never to use.

In regard to those instances where it seems as if it would be necessary to use instruments, I quote the following rules adopted by accoucheurs: 1. Meddlesome midwifery is always bad. 2. In no case need we interfere when the obstacles to be overcome can be overcome in a reasonable time by nature or without an operation. 3. Cases in which instruments are to be used are exceptions to the general rule, and no instrument should be used in a clandestine manner. 4. We should not have such an aversion to the use of instruments that we too long delay that assistance we have the power of affording with them.

PLACENTAL PRESENTATION.

PLACENTA PREVIA will never be treated by the nurse, but she should know its nature, know that it is this that causes unavoidable hemorrhage, and she should not fail to obtain a skillful physician early, to attend the case. The flooding is the necessary consequence of the dilatation of the os uteri, by which the connection between the placenta and uterus is separated, and the more the labor advances, the greater the disruption, and the more excessive the hemorrhage.

The woman usually passes through the early part of pregnancy without any sign that denotes the peculiar attachment, but the placenta can easily be distinguished from the membranes or coagulated blood as soon as the os uteri is a little opened. When a hemorrhage comes on from this cause the patient is never free from danger till she be delivered. Often the medical man is obliged to free the patient from imminent danger by artificial delivery, but I can conceive of no circumstance in which a *nurse* would be justified in turning for unavoidable hemorrhage.

Before, during, and after the delivery, the appliances used in other cases of hemorrhage may be used with some advantage, but I would hardly advise the nurse to do any thing before the doctor arrives.

ACCIDENTALHEMORRHAGE.

That form of FLOODING that arises from a partial and accidental separation of the placenta which occupies its usual position, must here be briefly referred to, as the nurse may be called on to do something in an emergency. The immediate cause of the flow is the separation of some portion of the placenta from the womb, and the laceration of the vessels. The hemorrhage is at first internal, is accompanied with dull pain at the spot where it takes place, it generally becomes external, it may or may not be attended with the discharge of coagula from the os uteri, and when the discharge commences it varies in quantity from a few ounces to an amount that is alarming. It is generally necessary to make a digital examination, to distinguish the accidental from the unavoidable hemorrhage.

Until the doctor arrives the patient should be kept in bed on a hard mattrass and very lightly covered with bed clothes. The temperature of the room should be kept very low, and nothing but cold water allowed.

The danger from hemorrhages that occur at or near the full period of utero gestation, may often be estimated by the absence or degree of pain, as well as from the quantity of the discharge. Hemorrhages are much more dangerous with sudden than with slow discharges of blood, and women are always in greater danger when they are not accompanied with pain.

Puerperal convulsions, whether of the hysteric, epileptiform, or apoplectic variety will always demand and almost always receive the prompt attention of the physician.

While the nurse is waiting for the doctor to arrive she might possibly administer a cathartic, thirty grains of bromide of potash, and an enema, but as a general rule she should not give anything. She might insert a wedge or roll of linen between the teeth to prevent injury to the tongue, and she should remove every thing out of the way, by striking against which, the patient might hurt herself.

CHAPTER I.
CAUSES OF DISEASE.

The causes of disease are spoken of by authors as predisposing, and exciting. By proximate cause of disease is meant the cause of the symptoms present; this cannot appropriately be dwelt upon here.

By exciting cause is meant the immediate cause of a disease, and the distinction from predisposing cause arises from the fact that when two persons are exposed to something injurious to the health, they may not be equally affected.

It has been said that if twenty persons undergo hardship and exposure from shipwreck, the effect of the wet and cold may be in one to cause catarrh, in another rheumatism, in a third pleurisy, in a fourth opthalmia, in another inflammation of the bowels, and fifteen may escape without any illness at all. A predisposing cause is defined to be anything whatever, which has had such an influence on the body as to have rendered it unusually susceptible to the exciting cause of the particular disease. In most cases the distinction is obvious, but it is sometimes difficult to say of a given cause whether it ought to be ranked among the predisposing or the exciting causes.

Disease is often warded off notwithstanding the presence of the exciting cause, when we ascertain and prevent the predisposing cause of it, and it may sometimes be averted in despite of strong predisposition, if we know and can guard against the agencies by which it is capable of being excited.

When we enumerate causes of disease we see among them many that under ordinary circumstances minister to life, health, and enjoyment; and I can hardly refer at all to the varying circumstances under which they become the medium of pain, disease and death. These circumstances are so various, so many of them are apt to be put in operation at the same time, and so little power have we of excluding them one after the other, so as to ascertain the exact efficiency of each, that our observation respecting their actual effects are open to much fallacy.

We cannot for instance in a given case estimate accurately the effect of impurities in the atmosphere such as organic and inorganic dust, nor the effect of differences in degree of its natural qualities such as extremes of heat and cold, sudden variations of temperature, excessive moisture or dryness, different electric conditions, differences of pressure, a deficiency of light, and the amount of ozone, &c.

OF HEAT AND COLD AS EXTERNAL AGENCIES CAUSING DISEASE.

The range of temperature compatible with human life is very great; men live in the hottest and the coldest climates, where the earth produces any sustenance for them. It requires more care to preserve life under intense cold than under intense heat. Tropical climates are thickly peopled where the thermometer ranges from 80° to 100° for a long time together. In arctic countries on the other hand where the thermometer sinks to 40° or 50° below zero, we still find inhabitants, but they are few and thinly scattered. It is probable that at a degree of temperature a little greater than that of the equator or a little less than that of the poles men would perish.

Man is capable of existing under certain circumstances for a short time, and enduring a much higher degree of heat than the general atmosphere attains in the hottest portions of the earth, but there are generally some deleterious effects from hot climates or continued hot weather.

The effect of HEAT is to stimulate the organic functions of the body, but when considerable heat is applied for some time together its effect is to cause languor and lassitude, want of energy, a disinclination for exertion both bodily and mental; it has a depressing effect generally upon the animal functions or the nervous system, and there are some forms of disease that are distinctly traceable to heat as a cause.

We all know the effect of hot weather in causing perspiration, and when the operation of high temperature is continued for some time it has a marked influence upon the liver, increasing the quantity of bile that is secreted, and altering its sensible qualities; this is sometimes followed by inflammation of the liver.

In this country those attacks of vomiting and diarrhœa which are so common towards the latter end of summer or in autumn are the effects of a succession of hot days. In tropical climates the morbific effects of external heat are still more conspicuous, tending to violent disorders of the stomach and intestines, and also to acute inflammation of the liver and to acute abscesses in that organ.

In these cases the heated atmosphere unduly stimulating the secreting function of the liver creates the predisposition to the disease, while the exciting cause of the inflammation may be exposure to cold.

There may be deleterious effects from exposure to cold where the climate is quite hot. For instance a man may after the heat occasioned by the employments of the day, undress and lie opposite a window, his shirt wet with perspiration, to enjoy the sea breeze at night, and though the thermometer may be as high as 80° he may have a sensation of cold. If there is real chilliness it may be deleterious.

Heat sometimes acts as an *exciting* cause of disease—it produces sunstroke, or it may produce an eruptive disease such as prickly heat, &c.

The effect of extreme COLD (I use the term cold in the popular acceptation), when its application is continued, is that of a sedative upon the organic functions. Though at first causing pain in the extremities, if continued it causes sleep or overpowering drowsiness. Before this complete stupor comes on there may be a blunting of the sensations and confusing of the intellect, giving to the person exposed to it, the appearance of one intoxicated. When persons in this state are suffered to sleep, and the operation of the cold continues, they become less and less sensible to external impressions until death closes the scene.

But the effect of cold upon the body within certain limits of intensity and duration is that of a tonic. When its refrigerating and sedative properties can be sufficiently counteracted by exercise and warm clothing, cold is stimulating, refreshing, and invigorating to mind and body, it clears and sharpens the faculties, bestows alacrity and cheerfulness of spirits, and may become a curative agent.

Yet exposure to cold is one of the most common causes of various complaints. As a rule it is true that there is danger from sudden vicissitudes of temperature, although the proposition requires limitation. No peril need attend a change from a hot to a cold temperature if the power to evolve heat inherent in the system be entire and active and persistent, not lessened by any of those circumstances which have the effect of weakening it, such as local disease, and fatigue. Cold is dangerous, not especially when the body is hot, but when it is cooling after being heated. At such times taking a large draught of cold water, or cooling the body suddenly some other way might cause death immediately; if not, an inflammation of some internal part of the body might arise.

Every thing that has the effect of weakening the system and so diminishing the power of evolving heat, favors the morbific effect of cold, and is a predisposing cause of disease. The most common of these debilitating circumstances are fasting, evacuations, fatigue, a last night's debauch, excess in venery, long watching, much study, and rest or inaction immediately after it, or after great exercise.

The faculty of evolving heat is weak in old persons and in the newly born, and these are often the victims of the power of cold.

The bad effects of cold depend very much upon the duration of the sensation. Even slight feelings of chilliness, if long protracted, are apt to terminate in some form of disease.

Cold is more likely to prove injurious when it is applied by a wind or currant of air, and the injurious operation of cold is augmented when it is accompanied with moisture—wetness is the worst way in which cold can be applied. The contact of wet or damp clothes with the skin, both increase and prolong the sensation of cold. A foggy atmosphere is more prejudicial than a clear one of the same temperature. While we are asleep, also, our power of resisting the effects of cold is diminished.

The power of habit enables a person to resist the effect of cold, and we may sometimes turn our knowledge of it to good account in gradually fortifying the system against the influence of cold that cannot be avoided. But we must not, while we fear to render our children effeminate by over care and much clothing, run into the opposite extreme and endanger their health by exposure. The process of hardening is doubly dangerous when it is attempted with children who were originally delicate, and should never be tried on any child or any person who is unsound, who shows any signs of present or approaching disease, or any marked predisposition to future, and especially to scrofulous disease.

An abiding sense of chilliness must never be permitted even when we are endeavoring to accustom a child to cold. If they can be kept in the cold air, and at the same time be kept feeling warm either by exercise, diversion of the mind, or by clothing, the result as regards the health is good.

The cold bath, and especially the shower bath, is a good means of fortifying the body against cold air. When we take a cold bath in the morning, if the sense of cold does not remain long, and is followed by a glow of warmth, the bath is sure to do good. If, however, after the bath we suffer headache, and continue to be chilly and languid or uncomfortable, it should at once be given up as useless and dangerous.

EFFECTS OF THE SEASON UPON HEALTH.

In this country, generally, catarrh and coughs and pectoral complaints of all kinds, are most apt to prevail in the winter and spring months, while bowel complaints are more numerous and distressing in the summer. The mucous membranes of the air passages sympathize with the skin under the agency of external cold; those of the stomach and intestines under that of heat.

The thoracic disorders which commence or grow worse in the winter are often fatal, and there are various other maladies that are aggravated by cold, so that the mortality of winter is greater than that of summer. Bowel complaints are more prevalent at the latter part of summer or early fall, when moderately cold days succeed a long period of hot weather, the high diurnal temperature being the predisposing cause, and the cold exciting or bringing on the disease.

I shall not refer to other causes of disease except to say that if two persons marry each other who have a hereditary predisposition to disease, their children, if they have any, will probably not be healthy.

CHAPTER II.
SYMPTOMS OF DISEASE, WITH INSTRUCTION TO NURSES.

Symptoms are the signs by which we know that disease is present. Every circumstance happening in the body of the sick person capable of being perceived by himself or others, which can be made to assist our judgment concerning the seat or nature of the disease, its probable course and termination or its proper treatment, is a sign or symptom.

These phenomena are the evidence upon which the whole art of the physician proceeds. It is important that the nurse should know how to note the symptoms, not only that she may know how and report to the doctor changes that occur in his absence, but that she may be able also to minister to those who are suddenly attacked with sickness, and to judge whether in cases of slight indisposition it is necessary to send for a physician.

By arranging and comparing symptoms, and by noting the circumstances under which they occur, the physician can distinguish the disease, and learn what are the indications of treatment—this belongs especially to him. But it is very important that a nurse should know how to note all changes as they occur, and sometimes it is best she should keep a written record of them. An important point in a trained or skillful nurse is that of her ability to observe accurately and describe intelligently what comes under notice in the absence of the physician. She should cultivate the habit of strict observation, and simple and truthful statement—neither deficient, exaggerated, or perverted, stating facts and not opinions.

Symptoms or phenomena which accompany disease may be *subjective*, those which are evident only to the patient, or *objective* which are observable by others. Both sorts of symptoms shed mutual light on each other, and as the statements of the patient are not always trustworthy, the nurse should be careful not to let anything pass unseen that can by vigilance be noted.

The following directions will help the nurse to cultivate the habit of observing symptoms:

Try to learn all you can of the previous history of the case; you will sometimes get information which the patient would not be likely to communicate to the doctor in person.

Note the patient's apparent age with any indications of disguised age, signs of weakness—whether corpulent or bloated; note any deformities, swellings or wounds, and notice the attitudes and expression of the countenance.

A sufferer instinctively takes THE POSITION most conducive to ease. When one lung is affected the patient lies on that side, that the healthy one may have the greater freedom of motion. When there is peritonitis (inflammation of the bowels), he lies on his back with his knees drawn up to relax the abdominal muscles. If there is colic alone he may lie on the abdomen, as pressure may relieve his pain. When a patient has been persistently on his back, if he turns onto his side it is a sign of improvement.

Inability to breathe termed ORTHOPNŒA, occurs in affections of the heart, and also in asthma. Lying quietly in bed is usually a favorable sign. Restlessness and slipping to the foot of the bed, in low stages of fever, are bad signs.

Of the uneasy, morbid symptoms, *pain* is the most important, and most common. Pain occurs in nearly all inflammations, and it may occur where there is no inflammation at all.

Bones, muscles, tendons, ligaments, the bladder, the kidneys, the uterus, all modify in a manner that is peculiar to themselves the pain that is produced by injury or disease. Such terms as the following are used to express a peculiar character of pain: It is said to be sharp, shooting, growing, burning, dull, heavy, tearing, and so on.

If pain is felt in any part when pressure is made upon it the heightened sensibility is called TENDERNESS, the part is said to be tender. A part may be both painful and tender, as it usually is if the pain continue for a time; it may be tender without being painful as it is usually, if pain continued for a time and then ceased.

Itching is an uneasy sensation allied to pain. It often affects the natural outlets of the body. It occurs about the rectum from the motions of little worms that nestle there, and other causes; and this itching of the rectum, and likewise of the pudendum, are distressing complaints, harassing the patient continually, preventing sleep and requiring medical treatment (F. 195). The tingling and pricking often felt in the windpipe, and provoking coughing, has some analogy to itching.

NAUSEA is sometimes a direct symptom of gastric disorder, at other times it is a very important indirect result of disease at some distance from the stomach. The nausea which is so troublesome to pregnant women, is an instance of a morbid sensation, sympathetic of irritation in a distant organ.

DIZZINESS or vertigo results sometimes from disease within the head, and sometimes it is the indirect result of disease of the stomach or of mere debility.

A sensation of sinking, sensations of weight and lightness, of drowsiness, tenesmus, strangury, heartburn, and various conditions of the special senses are mostly SUBJECTIVE SYMPTOMS.

One of the first symptoms of diabetis is a preternatural keenness of appetite, but in most diseases the appetite is lost or impaired or perverted.

THIRST is generally great in diabetis, and there is commonly considerable thirst in inflammatory complaints.

The above named symptoms are mostly subjective, but are accompanied by others that are objective, that show that the functions of certain parts are disturbed or suspended; and it is of especial importance to notice the PULSE, as this is a valuable guide in treating disease.

Each contraction of the heart sends out a wave which distends the blood vessels, and they by their contractility or elasticity carry it on through the entire arterial system. This periodical distention is the pulse.

The PULSE BEATS can be felt wherever an artery approaches the surface; it is usually taken and counted at the wrist; in children it can be best taken at the temporal artery during sleep.

To take the pulse accurately place two or three fingers on the artery making moderate pressure, and note particularly its frequency, its regularity, its forces and its fullness.

The RATE varies with varying circumstances. The average number of pulsations in a healthy adult is from 70 to 75, but there are some persons who, when they are quite well have a pulse of 80 or 90 to the minute, and there are others in whom it seldom rises above 60. It is usually more rapid in women than in men, is much more frequent in early life than in old age, and the average rate in a healthy child is 120.

In disease, the pulse may acquire a great degree of frequency. It may reach 150 or even 200, but in such cases it is generally feeble and can hardly be counted. Besides observing the frequency of the pulse, its character in other respects must be noted.

IRREGULARITY OF THE PULSE generally indicates disease, and there are two varieties of it. In most instances of irregular pulse, succeeding beats differ in length, force and character; in the other variety a pulsation is from time to time left out; the pulse is said to intermit.

In the DICROTIC PULSE a secondary wave or undulation can be felt. It is often met in typhoid fever, and an inexperienced person might be led to count double the number of beats.

Another important quality of the pulse is its hardness or compressibility. The hard pulse ordinarily, though not always, indicates inflammation. This hard pulse may be known by pressing pretty hard with one finger, while we observe with the others whether we arrest or abolish the pulse.

A pulse is said to be full or large if it is felt to strike a large portion of the finger; other departures from the normal standard are spoken of as soft, quick, or sharp, throbbing, bounding, thready, wiry, flickering, &c.

OF THE TEMPERATURE.

The normal standard of the temperature of a healthy person is 98.4°. There is some variation, and indeed a daily cycle of variations, so that in the morning it is 99 or at least 98½ and in the evening 97½, but the range is small, and if the variation is more than that, it is indicative of disease. There is only a deviation of about 15° within which life can be sustained; a temperature of more than 107° or less than 93° will almost certainly prove fatal.

Every mother who can, as well as every nurse, ought to own a clinical thermometer, as thereby she may detect the beginning of a disorder before there are other marked signs of indisposition. She should use it upon the first suspicion of a departure from health and frequently afterwards, until she knows that the temperature is normal. An increase, especially if beginning each day a little earlier, is a bad indication; a decrease from a high temperature each day is a sign of improvement. In pneumonia and generally in such disorders as are initiated with a chill, the rise is sudden and rapid.

In typhoid and some other fevers, the elevation is slight at first and gradually rises. The exacerbations and remissions or other deviations can only be recognized by taking the temperature frequently, and it should be taken at the same hour each day to exhibit the cycle of changes.

An irregularity of temperature in the course of a disease that has a regular type may indicate a complication, or it may depend upon local causes, such as constipation, bad air, &c. The decline of fever and of temperature may be gradual, or it may drop to a steady normal within a few hours.

Before using the thermometer the index must be thrown down to a point below the normal. Hold it with the bulb down and shake till it falls sufficiently.

The part (the axilla) should not have been exposed for washing for at least half an hour before taking the temperature, and it is a good precaution to keep the axilla (or mouth) closed for ten minutes before putting the bulb of the thermometer into it, and a little time may be saved by slightly warming the bulb in the hand before its introduction. If we are careful and see that the axilla is first dried from perspiration, and that the clothing is not in the way, and that the thermometer is held firmly in position a sufficient time, we may get a correct axillary temperature, unless in a very emaciated person. If taken in the mouth the lips must be closed during the process.

The rectum gives the most reliable temperature, and this method is employed for infants. The thermometer should be oiled and introduced for about two inches. Unless the presence of feces prevent, the thermometer will be half a degree higher than if taken in the axilla. It will sometimes take ten minutes or more to obtain the temperature, but some thermometers will do the work in less than five minutes.

THE RESPIRATION.

That respiration and circulation are intimately connected, and that whatever modifies the pulse usually effects the breathing is a fact generally known. That the proper performance of the function of every organ in the body depends somewhat upon proper respiration, is a fact not so generally known and recognized, and as this is an important topic we may properly here enlarge upon it.

By the muscular action of the diaphragm and intercostal muscles, and the consequent contractions and expansion of the lungs, the alternate inspirations and expirations are produced which we call breathing. The lungs are not completely filled and emptied by each respiration, and a certain amount of air remains stationary in them. Were this air which remains stationary constantly in a particular portion of the lungs, the same without change, we would derive no benefit from that portion of the lungs. Practically, however, it is believed that the additional supply breathed in and out is diffused through and alters the character of the whole.

A healthy adult ordinarily breathes about eighteen times per minute, taking in each time about twenty inches of air. It is said that it takes at this rate sixteen respirations to completely renovate the air. This is probably true of our ordinary breathing, but the renovation of the air depends upon our manner of breathing. It is possible for us to breath so that at one expiration we almost displace the air from every portion of our lungs, and then by a full, deep, prolonged inspiration, (throwing forward the chest, throwing back the shoulder, and keeping the body erect,) fill the lungs fully with air and thus not only change the air in our lungs, but change in some degree the character of our blood so as to increase its purity.

In order to test this let me ask anyone who is suffering from any slight indisposition, if it be headache, nausea, pains in different parts of the body, or any sickness, to try to breathe in this manner for half an hour, and observe if they do not feel better, being careful at the same time that the air breathed is good and pure. This point is of so much importance that I will refer to it again hereafter.

The character of the respiration is an important diagnostic symptom and should always be noted. The rate of respiration varies as does that of the pulse, but the former is partly under the control of the will. The respirations are more rapid in women than in men, in children than in adults; it is modified also by position, exertion, excitement, and other conditions. We may count the respirations by observing the rise and fall of the chest, but it is well to put our hand on the stomach where the motions may be felt.

Breathing is in man mostly abdominal, in woman mostly thoracic, but inflammation in the chest or abdomen will affect its character.

Dyspnœa, difficulty of breathing, arises when from any cause the amount of air entering the lungs does not correspond to the amount of blood sent by the heart for purification. The air may be unfit for its work, or disease in the lungs, or air passages may shut it out. Asphyxia results if the supply of air is in any way cut off.

OF THE AIR.

In this connection I will say to the nurse, give the patient pure air. Learn how indispensable this is to life, or health, or comfort; how indispensable to any person, and especially to the sick; how liable the air in the room is to be contaminated by the air breathed or expired by those in the room; by lights burning in the room; by exhalations from the bodies of the sick; by excreta left for a time in the room; by the inevitable floating dust from the floors and walls; from clothing, bedding, and furniture; and from the presence of organic matter in increased quantity, and of most deleterious quality in and around the sick.

A thousand feet of air space where the air is constantly renewed, is necessary for a healthy adult; a sick person should have two or three times as much, because with them there is increased susceptibility to draughts. Be very careful that the sick are not placed so that a direct current of air can blow on any part of the body, but either by the use of fans or in some other way the air must be renewed around their bed.

VENTILATION.

The problem to be solved is, how can fresh, pure air be best supplied? The inequalities of temperature within and without the room produces some natural ventilation, as this sets the air in motion and effects an exchange of air, if there are some apertures around the doors and windows.

This, however, is seldom sufficient, and artificial ventilation is often necessary. An open fire is a good apparatus for this purpose. The draught which it creates carries the air from the room up the chimney, while a fresh supply is drawn in to take its place. This supply should be from the outward air, or from an adjoining room in which the air is not contaminated.

The inlets and outlets for air should be of equal capacity, on opposite sides of the room, and of different heights to secure thorough ventilation. They should be as far as possible from the patient and from each other. In cold and damp weather great care is necessary to keep the air fresh and wholesome and at the same time to avoid chilling the patient. But even in cold weather the doors and windows may be thrown open for a minute at a time, if the patient is at the time protected by additional clothing.

However, during the night and in cold and wet weather, the principal supply of air will be from an adjoining room, air that is warmed, but it should be as pure as possible. When the weather is cold, and especially the latter part of the night, have more heat in the room and not less fresh air; if needed give your patient additional clothing and foot warmers.

The windows may be thrown open once or twice a day in cold weather, if the patient is protected by putting additional clothing on the bed, and using some sort of a screen, (an umbrella may be used for a screen), as a protection from the cold and direct draughts. But as the contamination of the air continues, the purification of it should be equally so, and some fresh air must constantly be admitted—some device used for the purpose. The window may be raised two or three inches and the aperture closed with a board, then the air will find admittance through the opening between the two sash; or when the window is raised three inches, a board six inches wide may be placed on the window sill a little inside of it; thus there will be an aperture both at the top and bottom of the lower sash. Or the upper sash may be lowered a little. The current of air which comes in (this is usually the lower one) should be directed upwards.

In the summer a lamp may be kept burning in the fireplace or grate; flues must in some way be kept heated or they will not draw. Stoves assist ventilation to some extent, but furnaces and radiators do not assist at all to ventilate, and the air is thereby especially dry. A pan of water may be kept boiling in the room, or perhaps merely setting on the stove, or a towel or two may be hung near a radiator and kept constantly wet; these will dampen the air by evaporation, and this is often necessary when the rooms are kept warm by artificial heat. About 66° is a proper temperature for a sick room in most cases, but 60° to 65° is suitable for fever cases; feeble and emaciated persons require a temperature of 70° to 75°.

Be careful to have the room warm when the patient is out of bed.

THE SYMPTOMS OF INFLAMMATION.

The ordinary symptoms which characterize inflammation may be known if we observe what takes place when an external part is injured. Let us suppose that a healthy man has a piece of glass stuck in his arm. He soon has pain, then redness in that part of his arm, then swelling, which is hard near the injury, and increases so that some swelling may be observed, though not so hard at a little distance, and the part is quite tender and hot.

These are the ordinary symptoms of inflammation: pain, redness, heat, and swelling, with tenderness that is manifested when the part is pressed.

If the inflammation increases there are signs of disorder in other parts of the body; the patient may be first chilly and feeble, then the skin may become hot and dry all over the body, the pulse fall hard and frequent, lassitude comes on with headache, perhaps pain in different parts of the body; he has also other symptoms of fever; is restless, sleeps ill, loses his appetite, his tongue becomes white, his mouth is dry, he is thirsty, the secretions of the body are diminished, has what is called inflammatory fever, or sympathetic fever, or pyrexia, the last term being now most generally used.

These phenomena, this inflammation, ends in two or three different ways. If measures have been taken for subduing the inflammation—in the supposed case of the arm—if the glass has been removed, it will probably happen that the symptoms above named will disappear. This is to end in what is called RESOLUTION.

When the inflammation goes on until pus is formed it is said to end in SUPPURATION. The symptoms grow more severe for several days, the swelling at length assumes a more pointed form, the skin in its centre begins to look white, and the swelling there gets softer; there is throbbing pain, perhaps the patient has chills or rigors; then when the swelling is cut open or the cuticle breaks a yellow creamlike fluid is poured out which is pus, and there is generally an abatement of the symptoms. If, however, the suppuration or discharge of pus continues for some time, other symptoms are manifested such as frequent shiverings, followed by flashes of heat which end in perspiration; this is HECTIC FEVER.

When the inflammation is still more intense it sometimes ends in MORTIFICATION, the part dies by the violence of the disease, the red color changing to a livid or purplish, or greenish black hue, the flesh losing its sensation and having an offensive odor.

Of course inflammation may be in an organ or structure that is internal, and we determine the seat of the disease, partly by the character of the pain. Sometimes the pain is sharp and piercing; this is its character generally in serous membranes such as the pleura or peritoneum (membranes covering the lungs and intestines.) There is less pain when the inflammation is in the mucous membrane, or in the parenchymatous structure of organs, such as the lungs, liver, and spleen.

There is generally an aggravation of pain upon pressing a part that is inflamed. Pain caused by air distending the bowels and stretching the nerves may be relieved by pressure. Spasmodic contractions of the muscles will cause pain without much tenderness.

OF HEAT AS A SYMPTOM OF INFLAMMATION.

The temperature of an inflamed part exceeds that which belongs to it in health. In inflammation as in fever, it has been known to rise to 107°. The increase of heat depends upon an influx of arterial blood, and therefore of oxygen into the part. There is probably always some increase of heat, though it may not always be noticed in every case of inflammation.

There is more REDNESS than is natural in a part that is inflamed. There is more blood than usual in the vessels that carry red blood, and the red blood enters into the small vessels where the red particles cannot commonly be seen. All the minute vessels seem to be enlarged. The redness often remains sometime after the inflammation has ceased.

The degree of SWELLING in different cases depends partly on the nature and structure of the part affected and partly on the intensity of the inflammation; in some instances there is so little that it is not appreciable.

Almost all the swelling results from the presence of matters thrown into the inflamed part. In the central hard portion the hardness is to be ascribed to an effusion into the areolar tissue of it, of a fluid which is transparent at first, afterwards becoming opaque, called coagulable lymph. Serum is effused into the areolar tissue of the softer swelling at the circumference.

ŒDEMA, DROPSY, ANASARCA.

Even under moderate inflammation some amount of effusion takes place into the texture or from the surface of a part. This effusive serous fluid called also serosity, resembles and probably is the scrum of the blood. When this passes into the areolar structure of a part it is called œdema, (though this is not always by inflammation) and if the serosity passes out extensively over the body, the disease is called anasarca or general dropsy.

If a considerable amount of this serous fluid is poured out in a short time from the peritoneum, it is a form of ascites or abdominal dropsy. If it is thus poured into the pleura it causes apnœa, or difficulty of breathing, and requires aspirating.

CHAPTER III.
DIAGNOSIS OF DISEASES IN CHILDREN, EARLY TREATMENT, &C.

It is not often that a correct diagnosis can be made of a disease by a single symptom, but there are marked and characteristic symptoms which indicate some diseases in children with considerable certainty.

A strongly marked nasal or palate sound in the child's cry indicates an abscess behind the pharynx. When this nasal tone is heard we should palpate with the finger on the throat to ascertain the degree of soreness.

A long drawn, ten times lengthened, loud sounding expiration with normal inspiration, and no dyspnœa is sufficient for the diagnosis of CHOREA MAJOR (St. Vitus dance.)

A high thoracic continually sighing inspiration, the upper part of the thorax doing the work of breathing, and with a sighing or groaning sound, shows the commencement of HEART WEAKNESS, CARDIAC PARALYSIS OR FATTY DEGENERATION OF THE HEART, and will probably be followed by such symptoms as cyanosis, coldness of the extremities, &c.

Strongly marked diaphragmatic expiration accompanied by a fine, high whistling sound, points to BRONCHIAL ASTHMA. This sound, however, resembles that made in croup. If there is a pause between the end of expiration and the beginning of inspiration, croup may be excluded.

Sleepiness, lasting twenty-four to thirty-six hours, occurring without fever or other disturbance to account for it, is an initial symptom of MENINGITIS, though it might be caused by narcotics or uremia.

A prominent, firm fontanelle means increase in quantity of the contents of the cranium-exudation of some sort. It cannot be caused by fullness of the vessels alone if it is firm and resisting. We know that we have cerebral disease with DROPSY or exudation (Hydrocephalus).

When the fontanelle is deeply sunken, it points to loss of blood or other nutritive juices, as in cholera, &c.

A sharp, shrill cry, accompanied by an expression of fright or great anxiety, and occurring about an hour after the child has fallen asleep, is the only symptom of the "ALP"—night terrors, sudden awaking from bad dreams.

Periodical crying, lasting from five to ten minutes, should always make us think of spasm of the bladder or PAINFUL URINATIONS.

Violent crying at stool with fear of the act, and general avoidance of it, points to FISSURE OF THE ANUS, and is usually accompanied with constipation.

A violent cry full of pain and almost continuous, with the throwing about of the head on the pillow and grasping it with the hands, means OTITIS or EARACHE.

Weakness or immobility of the child, after a comparatively slight or short illness, points to SPINAL PARALYSIS.

Delayed ossification of the cranial bones is an early sign of RICKETS, as is crying continued for weeks (increased on touch of the extremities), accompanied with fever and incessant sweating.

Vomiting of all kinds of food continued for weeks in children of closed cranium but with large cranial measurements, when there is no fever, pain, idiopathic disease, or a cerebral tumor, indicates chronic HYDROCEPHALUS with an acute onset.

Congestion of the cheeks in children, excepting in cases of cachexia and chronic disease, indicates an INFLAMMATION or a febrile condition.

Congestion of the face, ears and forehead of short duration, strabismus with febrile reaction, oscillation of the iris, irregularity of the pupil with falling of the upper lids, indicates a brain affection.

Enlargement of the spongy portions of the bones indicates RICKETS.

A thick and purulent secretion between the eyelids may indicate great PROSTRATION of the general powers.

Passive congestion of the conjunctival vessels indicates approaching DEATH.

Long continued lividity, as well as lividity produced by excitement or exercise, the respirations continuing normal, are indices of FAULT IN THE FORMATION OF THE HEART, or great blood vessels.

A temporary lividity indicates the existence of a grave acute disease, especially of the respiratory organs.

Irregular muscular movements, which are partly under the control of the will, indicates the existence of CHOREA (St. Vitus dance).

The contraction of the eyebrows, together with a turning of the head and eyes to avert the light, is a sign of cephalalgia (headache).

When the child holds its hand upon its head, or strives to rest the head upon the bosom of the mother or nurse, it may be suffering from ear disease.

When the fingers are carried to the mouth, and there is besides great agitation apparent, and when it turns its head from one side to another, there is probably some obstruction or some abnormal condition of the larynx.

A feeble and plaintive cry indicates a trouble in the abdominal regions.

If the respiration is intermittent but accelerated, there is capillary bronchitis. In bronchitis the cough is clear and distinct.

A hoarse and rough cough is indicative of true CROUP. When the cough is suppressed and painful, there is PNEUMONIA or PLEURISY.

In diseases of the stomach, liver or bowels we have usually a coated tongue; a white tongue indicates FEBRILE disturbance or some THROAT trouble; a brown moist tongue, INDIGESTION; a brown dry tongue, DEPRESSION, BLOOD POISONING or TYPHOID FEVER; a red moist tongue, INFLAMMATORY FEVER; a broad, pale flabby tongue accompanies a DROPSICAL CONDITION of the system; a tremulous, moist and flabby tongue indicates FEEBLENESS, NERVOUSNESS; a pale flabby tongue which shows the pressure of the teeth, a generally relaxed condition of the system; the irritable or strawberry tongue with its red papilla, points to an irritated stomach, and is met with in SCARLET FEVER; a furred and dry tongue is indicative of VIOLENT LOCAL INFLAMMATION; if afterwards clean, red and dry, protracted INFLAMMATORY FEVER.

Wheezing cough and wheezing breathing indicates ASTHMA; dull, heavy aching pain at the base of the chest, ACUTE BRONCHITIS; urgent desire to go to stool, DYSENTERY; diminished secretion of urine, INFLAMMATORY and FEBRILE DISORDERS; cold hands and feet, NERVOUS DISEASES and low states of the blood.

In general, the diagnosis of diseases of children is easy if we simply compare the objective symptoms with those which should obtain in a healthy child of the same age. But we must remember that with children symptoms which appear very grave are often evanescent, and on the other hand the indications of very serious disease may be disregarded on account of their natural vivacity and recuperative powers. In each case each child should be studied by itself considering its antecedents, its peculiarities, its surroundings, and its relations to them.

The mother has the best chance to know these; she sees the child when awake and asleep, when dressed and undressed; she knows its history, what has been its diet, what her own health has been, her own habits, her surroundings and occupations, and whether there may or may not have been anything to cause sickness of the child in her own toils or trials. The nurse and the mother should note all the facts, for their own guidance and for the guidance of the physician if he is called.

EARLY TREATMENT OF INFANTILE DISEASES.

Very few of the symptoms heretofore mentioned can be neglected with impunity. While some cases of sickness may be left to the powers of nature to restore health, others require judicious early treatment, and a physician should be called. We should generally enjoin rest, but we should act by our medicines to meet every positive indication.

We are the assistants of nature; we must act by removing the causes where they can be reached; we must relieve pain, but we must not by officious kindness do too much and interfere with the natural return to health. Remember that drugs are not all powerful, that time, rest, diet and numberless little things are the means by which we aid in the fight against disease.

It is an excellent plan not to continue medicine too long. Place the child on the road to health and see if it will not with a little supervision improve—still, however, using proper rest, diet, &c.

But as the apparently trifling symptoms of to-day may become the full fledged attack of to-morrow, we must pay attention to every untoward symptom. Parents are liable to be unnecessarily scared, and afterwards go to the other extreme and neglect calling a physician until serious injury has occurred.

I will here give you a few aphorism and general rules: Treatment of the sick should be according to the patient as well as according to the disease. Adult males are not so sensitive as females; young children, whether male or female, are sensitive, tender and excitable, and alive to every irritation.

But young children differ in their constitution, and some have peculiarities or idiosyncracies so that medicines of ordinary activity act very powerfully or even violently.

Small children are always sensitive to the action of medicine, and small doses only are required for them. And in consequence of the activity of the vital powers, and the quickness and force of the circulation, there is a remarkable susceptibility to inflammatory action, disease sometimes running on rapidly to organic and incurable mischief.

In treating children employ the mildest remedies at first, and aid their action by regimen. When an emergency demands, use those articles which experience has shown to have power to meet such an emergency. Exhibit such medicine in the minimum dose and increase or repeat until the desired effect is produced. Be very careful not to fill the child with nostrums for some imaginary ill, lest you thereby make it ill. Always remember that the first step in treatment is to change the conditions which produced the disease—remove the cause and assist nature to repair the injury.

CHAPTER IV.
TREATMENT OF INFLAMMATION IN ITS INCIPIENT STAGES.

Usually the nurse or the mother does not treat disease, or administer medicine except under the direction of a physician, and it is not always necessary for her to know the principles that guide in their administration, or why particular medicines are given. But it is sometimes necessary for the nurse or mother to decide what shall be done, and to act before the doctor can be consulted. Accidents and emergencies occur, distress and sickness may suddenly attack some member of a family at any time, and little ailments are complained of every day by some of them; the question arises, what shall be done?

It is not necessary every time to send for the physician, and he cannot at a moment's notice be obtained. For many ailments the mother prescribes, and many times the early and judicious use of medicines or regimen not only relieves present suffering, but also prevents the developement of serious, and protracted and dangerous maladies. This is especially true in regard to incipient inflammation, and I shall here speak particularly of its treatment.

What has heretofore been said about inflammation gives us some guide to enable us to know whether the case calling for our care is one of an inflammatory character. If the pulse is full and hard and a little more frequent than usual, and there is restlessness and some pain we may conclude that there is IRRITATION that precedes inflammation at least, before such symptoms as depression, chilliness followed by heat, headache, a furred tongue, loss of appetite, and apparent weakness come on. But if any of these symptoms are present we should search for the cause. Perhaps if the inflammation is external we shall be able to ascertain what produces the trouble. In every case we ought to know the cause if possible, as we thus have more clear indications for treatment.

But we may use the sedative treatment in all cases where these symptoms come on in a person who has previously been healthy. Of course you will not bleed—that, if done at all, should be done by the doctor. But all sources of irritation ought to be removed, so that the patient may enjoy perfect quiet; the sick room should be ventilated, and kept at the temperature of about 60°; let the diet be light; allow ice and cold water freely, and if there is much febrile excitement use sedatives and saline refrigerants. The best sedative is veratrum viride, and the following is a convenient way of administering it: Drop 30 drops of the fluid extract of veratrum in 30 teaspoonfuls of water and give 1 teaspoonful every two hours. To adult subjects if there is considerable fever two drops of the extract, or two teaspoonfuls of the diluted preparation may be given at first and the dose may be repeated in an hour, but it will not be best to continue such large doses. Aperients may be given if there are fecal accumulations in the bowels. Although quinine is a tonic, six to ten grains of it are sometimes given with good effect in a case of inflammation.

Opium is a good remedy judiciously given; one dose (1 grain for an adult) is good in a case of catarrh or cold; successive doses are necessary in a case of peritonitis or enteritis, but this should be given on a physician's advice. It acts probably by quieting the nerves—by sustaining the faltering action of the heart, and by keeping the inflamed part at rest. Sometimes cold, and sometimes hot applications are made to inflamed parts, and it is said that the sensations of the patient are the best criterion of their usefulness. Except, however, in cases of inflammation of the brain, and perhaps even then, I think that hot applications are the best. When we wish to promote suppuration hot fomentations should be applied.

Counter irritants relieve inflammation of the deeper parts by drawing the circulating fluid and the nervous energy to the surface. The milder kinds called rubefacients, produce merely local warmth and redness; these may often be used advantageously. Mustard applied so as to redden the skin is generally useful.

Vesicants, epispastics, or blistering agents are safe appliances but they are distressing, and their use may be deferred until a physician advises them.

I have said that the diet should be light while the pulse is hard and full. Afterwards when the pulse is natural, or if it becomes irregular or small, good broths or other nutrients are to be given, milk, cream, and even raw eggs may be administered. In general food should not be pressed upon a patient.

OF TOPICAL APPLICATIONS FOR INFLAMMATION.

I have mentioned counter irritants and I think it best at this time to advert to all the various topical applications, irritating, soothing and protective, and to give such instructions as I can in regard to them.

Counter irritants are frequently applied over or near the seat of the disease, and often also at a remote part to obtain what is called revulsive action. In both instances, however, their action may be revulsive. If applied to the thorax or chest, for example in a case of pneumonia, the cuticle to which it is applied is almost as remote from the lung by the way of the circulation, as is the cuticle of the wrist or ankle. But practically a sinapism may be very useful applied at either place—possibly more useful if applied over the seat of the inflammation, because there is a sympathy between the parts—they may be used very beneficially in domestic medication.

In a few succeeding pages I give some directions to the nurse who acts under the doctor's orders.

Ammoniacal liniments, and other washes and embrocations that are sufficiently irritating to produce redness when rubbed on the skin, should be rubbed on briskly so as to produce considerably increased circulation in the capillaries, &c. One of the most commonly used rubefacients is mustard. To make a mustard plaster, or sinapism, take one part of powdered mustard, and about three times the quantity of flour and mix into a paste with tepid water, and spread it evenly between two pieces of thin muslin. As hot water or vinegar weakens the active principle of mustard, tepid water is best, even if it seems cold when applied to the patient. Good sinapisms are conveniently made also by doubling brown paper several thicknesses, wetting it and sprinkling on the mustard alone.

The mustard must not be left on long enough to vesicate; usually it should be taken off within half an hour (or moved,) except when applied to the soles of the feet, when they may commonly be left on for several hours. Their action must be carefully watched upon an insensible or delirious patient, or a little child. In mixing the plaster for children glycerine may be used, and then the plaster may remain on longer. Confine in place by a bandage. If the patient complain of the burning or smarting after the plaster is removed, dust the part with starch or fine flour, or dress with vaseline to exclude the air.

You may make a cayenne pepper plaster in the same way that a mustard plaster is made, or you may sprinkle pepper upon a thin slice of pork. This makes good draughts for children and may be useful sometimes for sore throat if applied to the neck. But capsicum plasters, &c., can be bought at the drug store. In the country it is generally convenient to obtain and apply horse radish leaves; these are good rubefacients. In order to produce immediate VESICATION I have known a doctor to heat an iron spoon until it was sufficiently hot, and then rub it over a small space of skin; and a small blister may be quickly made by saturating a bit of cotton with hartshorn, putting it in a top thimble and applying it to the skin to remain seven or eight minutes. But the agent most commonly used to produce vesication is the CANTHARIDEAL PLASTER. If you are to produce a blister with this, the part should first be washed and dried, shaved if there is any hair upon it, then if you wish the blister to rise soon wet the plaster and also the skin with vinegar; apply, and secure the plaster in place by a bandage. Most commonly it will rise in from four to eight hours, but without waiting for it to rise fully you may remove the plaster and apply a poultice which will produce the desired effect. Do not tear the skin in taking the plaster off. When the blister is well raised make a slight incision or two for the escape of serum, and dress with vaseline or tallow. This is the usual way, but in some cases the physician may direct differently, perhaps may leave the blister undisturbed and allow the fluid to be reabsorbed.

Strangury and congestion of the kidneys sometimes follow the prolonged use of cantharides; to prevent this, it is sometimes recommended that tissue paper be well oiled and interposed between the plaster and skin. And as camphor corrects the action of cantharides upon the bladder, it is recommended that in case of a child particularly, a solution of camphor in ether be sprinkled upon the plaster. If a blister is applied to a young child, it should be carefully watched and not allowed to remain too long. In two or three hours the skin will be well reddened, and the plaster may be removed and a poultice applied.

TINCTURE OF IODINE is sometimes applied as a counter irritant, but several coats and repeated applications are necessary to produce a blister.

Local stimulation can be obtained from bits of cantharideal plaster kept on for an hour or two, and removed or changed before the point of vesication is reached. The same effect follows the rapid passage of a hot flat iron over a piece of brown paper or flannel laid upon the skin. It is generally best that the flannel should be wet first; and should an emergency arise when from hemorrhage or some other cause there is danger of immediate collapse, the application of heat in this way may rouse the sufferer and prevent immediate death. This or the actual cautery is sometimes used to relieve lumbago, or rheumatism. If you have thereby a slight burn, you may dress it in a solution of bicarbonate of soda and cover from air with rubber tissue.

If a SETON is inserted in the skin, the silk should be moved daily and the matter well cleared out.

WET CUPS are applied to relieve congestion and to abstract blood, the skin being first scarified.

DRY CUPPING is most practiced for the relief of pain and to draw the blood away from an inflamed organ. Small tumblers may be used in the absence of cupping glasses, if the edges are smooth. When you apply the cups have at hand also a lamp, a saucer of alcohol, a bit of sponge or a wad of lint fastened to the end of a stick. Have the cups perfectly dry, dip the sponge in the alcohol which you will ignite from the lamp, (they being near the patient), and let it burn for an instant in the inverted glass, then withdraw and extinguish it, and rapidly place the cup over the intended spot. As the heated air in the glass condenses in cooling, the skin will be forcibly sucked up, and the blood drawn towards the surface. Each cup will remain on from three to five minutes. Do not attempt to apply them to a bony and irregular surface, and be very careful not to burn the patient by getting the edges of the glass too hot. To remove the cup press with the finger close to the cup so that air will be admitted.

WET CUPPING will be attended to by the physician, who will provide the scarificator, and adhesive straps. See that plenty of soft towels are provided.

There are two varieties of LEECHES used in this country, the American and the foreign. The latter differs from the former in having five or six stripes down its back instead of three, and it will draw from five to six times its own weight of blood as it is larger and more voracious than the American variety.

The domestic variety is sometimes preferred for children, as it will draw a sufficient amount of blood usually. Leeches should not be applied over any large vessel, and preferably should be over a bony surface where pressure can be made to stop the blood if it continues to run. The leech should not be handled, it may be washed and dried in the folds of a towel.

To induce them to bite, the part to which they are to be applied must be perfectly clean, and it may be best to pick or scratch the skin so that the leech has first a taste of blood; or you may put the leech in a wine glass, test tube, leech glass, or small bottle filled with water; cover with a cord and invert over the place; hold it close and slip out the paper. The leech will then probably take hold and the glass can be taken off, and the water absorbed by a towel. If one is to be applied inside the mouth or nostril, put a thread through its tail to prevent its being swallowed. If such an accident should occur have the patient drink freely of salt and water, and induce vomiting.

If the leech seems sluggish when applied stroke it gently with a dry towel. When full it will drop off. If you wish to take them off sooner, do not remove by force, but put a little salt on their heads. If the bleeding from the orifice continues too long it may be checked by a compress of lint, an application of ice, or by touching with nitrate of silver, or carbolic acid. Leeches not used may be kept in a jar of water with sand in the bottom, and a perforated cover, or it may be covered with a linen cloth. The water in which they are kept should be changed twice a week in winter and oftener in summer. Salt will make a leech disgorge the blood with which it is filled, but if kept afterwards it is liable to be diseased, and to cause disease in those that are with it.

By FOMENTATIONS or stupes is commonly meant the application of flannels or towels wet with hot water or some medicinal decoction. If hot water only is used, they are a convenient means of applying warmth and moisture, but they require constant attention, needing to be changed every ten or fifteen minutes. They are chiefly of use in relieving pain and inflammation, and in promoting suppuration when that is desirable.

Two pieces of flannel should be at hand each doubled to the desired size; they are to be saturated with boiling water and wrung out dry as possible. To wring it out without scalding one's fingers, put it inside a towel, and this may be made with a hem at the end so that a stick can be thrust through it. Wring the flannel so dry that it will not make the bed or bed clothing wet. Cover with oiled muslin a little larger than the fomentation, and over that lay some dry flannel or cotton. If the stupe is put on hot, and frequently changed, it derives or draws blood towards the skin, and is often useful in relieving spasm and pain; and the continued use of them prevents suppuration. Medicaments are sometimes added to make them more irritant or sedative; then they are not changed so often, but they must not be allowed to get cold. After the fomentations are discontinued, carefully wipe the parts dry to which they have been applied, and cover with a warm, dry flannel.

I subjoin a few useful fomentations in which decoctions or medicines are used.

1. Add one ounce muriate of ammonia and two ounces spirits of camphor to 1 quart of boiling water just before dipping the flannel into it.

2. For a fomentation to the bowels, chest, &c., of a child, take 1 oz. paragoric, 1 oz. Jamaica ginger, and 4 ozs. hot water.

3. Twenty drops spirits turpentine may be sprinkled over each stupe, but be careful about blistering the skin or making a sore.

4. A decoction of chamomile flowers, hops, or conium, may be used for the fomentation instead of water.

5. Twenty drops or more of laudanum may be dropped over each stupe. This might soothe pain without causing stupor.

POULTICES, like stupes, are means of applying warmth and moisture. If applied early, it is believed they may prevent the formation of pus, as they bring about a resolution of the inflammation. When suppuration has commenced they facilitate the passage of matter to the surface, and lessen the extent of the disease. When applied to an inflamed part or swelling they should extend over considerable surrounding surface, but for a suppurating wound they should be but little larger than the opening.

Avoid putting them on very hot in a case of paralysis and also upon children, though they should be applied quite hot usually.

To make BREAD POULTICES pour boiling water on slices of bread without crust, simmer a few minutes, then beat up the bread quickly and spread it upon a piece of muslin previously cut of the desired size, leaving about two inches of margin upon each side. Then put on the poultice some lard or oil or vaseline to keep it from getting dry and hard, and to make it less likely to stick. It will be well to put on it a cover of thin muslin or mosquito netting, or tulle, or illusion, and then fold over like a broad hem the edges of both the covers. The poultice should be evenly spread about a quarter of inch in thickness and may be carried to the patient on a small tray or board, and if you are changing the poultice you should also have a small basin to carry away the old ones. After applying the poultice cover with some impervious material (oiled muslin or rubber cloth) to keep in the heat. Such a poultice as this will keep warm for five or six hours, but it should not be allowed to become cold and hard. Milk should not be used in making poultices as it quickly sours.

POULTICES ARE MADE OF VARIOUS MATERIALS. Flax seed meal, starch, powdered slippery elm, Indian meal, and oat meal are used. They should all be made of such a consistence that they will be tenacious as possible, and should have at least a little oil on them to prevent their getting dry.

For PUTRID SORES some disinfectant solution may be used instead of water in making the poultice, such as a weak solution of chlorinated soda.

YEAST POULTICES are used to hasten the separation of gangrenous sloughs. Mix six ounces of yeast with the same quantity of water at blood heat. Stir in fourteen ounces of wheat flour and let it stand near the fire until it rises. Apply while fermenting, or, "Take of wheat flour a pound, yeast half a pint, mix, and expose the mixture to a gentle heat until it begins to rise."

The following are old officinal forms for poultices:

ALUM CATAPLASM. Take the whites of two eggs, of alum a drachm, shake them together so as to form a coagulum. (A common mode of preparing the alum poultices is to rub the whites of two eggs briskly in a saucer with a lump of alum till the liquid coagulates.) The curd produced by coagulated milk with alum is sometimes used as a substitute. The alum cataplasm is sometimes employed in incipient or chronic opthalmia as an astringent application. It is placed over the eye enveloped in folds of cambric or soft linen.

CATAPLASM CARBONIS LIGNI. Take a sufficient quantity of wood charcoal red hot from the fire, and having extinguished it by sprinkling dry sand over it, reduce it to very fine powder and incorporate in the simple cataplasm in a tepid state. Charcoal recently prepared has the property of absorbing those principles upon which the offensive odor of putrefying, animal substance depends. In the form of poultice it is an excellent application to foul and gangrenous ulcers, correcting their fetor and improving the condition of the sore. It should be frequently renewed.

Conium Cataplasm. Take of extract of poison hemlock (conium) two ounces, water a pint. Mix and add of bruised flax seed sufficient to produce a proper consistence. This cataplasm may be advantageously employed as an anodyne in cancerous, scrofulous, and other painful ulcers, but its liability to produce narcotic effects in consequence of the absorption of the active principle of the hemlock must not be overlooked.

Sometimes a bag is made to contain a poultice, and such a bag should be used if we desire to apply a large poultice to the chest or abdomen. One can be made for the breast and for the back at the same time, and two straps over the shoulder may unite them. A hop poultice is a thin bag loosely filled with hops and wrung out of hot water.

Dry fomentations are sometimes employed. Thin bags filled with heated sand, ashes, salt, bran, or hops are used, to keep the heat applied to the skin; and to warm the feet and quicken the circulation in the extremities, hot bricks, bottles filled with water, &c., are applied. These should be rolled in hot flannel or at least enveloped in something.